Airedale **NHS**

NHS Trust

Library & Information Services

KEY QUESTIONS IN SURGICAL CRITICAL CARE

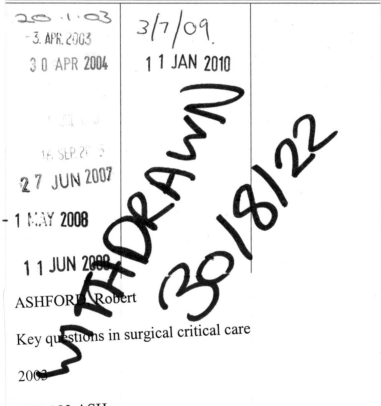

KEY QUESTIONS IN SURGICAL CRITICAL CARE

by

Mr Robert U. Ashford MRCS(Glasg)

Specialist Registrar in Trauma & Orthopaedics
York District Hospital
Yorkshire Deanery
UK

Dr T. Neal Evans FRCA

Specialist Registrar in Anaesthesia
Oxford Radcliffe Hospitals
Oxford Deanery
UK

Dr R. Andrew Archbold MRCP

Specialist Registrar in Cardiology
London Chest Hospital
London Deanery (North)
UK

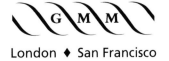

London ◆ San Francisco

www.greenwich-medical.co.uk

© 2003

Greenwich Medical Media Limited
137 Euston Road, London
NW1 2AA

870 Market Street, Ste 720
San Francisco, CA 94102

ISBN 1 84110 0927

First Published 2003

Typeset by Mizpah Publishing Services, Chennai, India
Printed by The Alden Group Ltd, Oxford

Distributed by Plymbridge Distributors Ltd and
in the USA by Jamco Distribution

Contents

Preface

Postgraduate surgical examinations take the form of multiple-choice questions, *viva voce* examinations and clinicals. In all the Royal Colleges, a key component of the first two of these sections is critical care. This book is a companion to *Surgical Critical Care*, by Robert Ashford and Neal Evans, published by Greenwich Medical Media Ltd in 2001, and examines all aspects of the subject that may be assessed.

This book is split into two sections: multiple-choice questions and *viva* topics. Based upon the syllabus of the Royal College of Surgeons of England, each of these two sections is sub-divided into the same six sections as *Surgical Critical Care.* Each answer is cross-referenced to specific pages in *Surgical Critical Care* (using the SCC icon) as well as being elaborated upon.

The multiple-choice questions are of a multiple true/false type. Marking should be in the form of the examination you are sitting. Remember some of the Royal Colleges employ negative marking, which is designed to prevent the candidate from guessing. The *viva* topics are questions typical of those you may be asked in the examination.

This book does not aim to be a definitive textbook for the MRCS examination. It is designed as a revision aid and to stimulate self-assessment.

Good luck!

R.U.A.
T.N.E.
R.A.A.
October 2002

The Examination

Whilst the Royal Colleges are working towards a unified MRCS examination, this is not yet in place. The Royal Colleges therefore have differing examination formats. Critical care is not specifically included in the clinical section of the examinations, therefore this is not discussed. As with all examinations, the format may change and candidates are advised to check the latest regulations with the relevant college.

England – MRCS

Two MCQ Papers: Core and Systems. Each paper consists of 65 MCQs and 60 EMQs to be answered in two and a half hours. Critical care is tested principally in Paper 1. Multiple true/false MCQs not negatively marked.

Three *Viva Voce* examinations each of 20 minutes: Anatomy, Physiology and Pathology. 10 minutes of Basic Science and 10 minutes of Clinical Surgery. Critical Care is examined for 10 minutes in the physiology viva.

Edinburgh – MRCS(Ed)

Two MCQ Papers: Core Syllabus and Systems Syllabus. Negatively marked.

Three *Viva Voce* examinations each of 20 minutes: Critical Care, Principles of Surgery, Clinical Surgery & Pathology.

Glasgow – MRCS(Glasg)

Two MCQ Papers: Core and Systems. 2 hours for each paper. Each paper is a combination of MCQs and EMQs. MCQs are multiple true/false and not negatively marked. Both papers must be sat the first time of entry.

Two *Viva Voce* examinations covering: Applied Anatomy, Operative Surgery & Principles of Surgery, Surgical Physiology & Critical Care and Applied Pathology & Bacteriology. 30 minutes each divided into the two sections. Critical Care forms a major part of the physiology viva.

Ireland – AFRCSI

Two MCQ Papers: Paper 1 is a Basic Sciences Paper: This is a true/false paper, which is 2 hours long. There are 30 five-part questions: 10 each in Anatomy, Physiology and Pathology. This paper will be negatively marked. Paper 2 is the Clinical Surgery Paper: This is a 2-hour paper consisting of 24 questions with 5 stems in each question. The second paper will be non-negatively marked. Minimum pass rate is 60%.

The *Viva Voce* examination consists of three 20-minute orals. The subjects are: Principles of Operative Surgery & Surgical Anatomy, Critical Care,

Surgical Emergencies & Applied Physiology, Surgical Management & Principles of Pathology. This College expects candidates to have a high level of knowledge of basic sciences. Therefore, each of these orals will include basic science examiners. Each marked out of 100, minimum to pass 180 out of 300.

There are a number of conventional terms applied to the examinations. These are outlined below:

Characteristic, predominantly, reliably	The feature is present in more than 90% of cases
Typically, frequently, commonly, usually	The feature is present in more than 60% of cases
Often, tends to	The feature is present in more than 30% of cases

Similarly, for percentages, a precise figure (e.g. 2.5%) means exactly that, whereas a round figure (e.g. 20%) allows a little either way ($\pm$5%).

As with all examinations, **read the question properly**.

List of Abbreviations

ABC	Airway, Breathing and Circulation
ABE	Actual base excess
ABG	Arterial blood gas
ACE	Angiotensin converting enzyme
ADH	Anti-diuretic hormone
AF	Atrial fibrillation
AHF	Acute hepatic failure
AIS	Abbreviated injury score
ALI	Acute lung injury
ALS	Advanced life support
AP	Antero-posterior
APACHE	Acute physiology and chronic health evaluation
APTT	Activated partial thromboplastin time
ARDS	Adult respiratory distress syndrome
ARF	Acute renal failure
ATN	Acute tubular necrosis
AXR	Abdominal X-ray
BAE	Bronchial artery embolisation
BLS	Basic life support
BMI	Body mass index
BMR	Basal metabolic rate
BSD	Brainstem death
BUN	Blood urea nitrogen
CABG	Coronary artery bypass grafting
CC	Closing capacity
CKMB	Creatinine kinase MB isoenzyme
CMV	Controlled mandatory ventilation/Cytomegalo virus
CNS	Central nervous system
CO	Cardiac output
COHb	Carboxyhaemoglobin
COPD	Chronic obstructive pulmonary disease
CPAP	Continuous positive airway pressure
CPB	Cardiopulmonary bypass
CPP	Cerebral perfusion pressure
CSF	Cerebrospinal fluid
CT	Computed tomography
CVP	Central venous pressure
CVS	Cardiovascular system
CXR	Chest X-ray
DC	Direct current
DIC	Disseminated intravascular coagulation
DO_2	Oxygen delivery

DPG	Diphosphoglycerate
DPL	Diagnostic peritoneal lavage
DVT	Deep vein thrombosis
EBV	Epstein-Barr virus
ECF	Extracellular fluid
ECG	Electrocardiogram
EDRF	Endothelium-derived relaxant factor
EDTA	Ethylene diamintetraacetic acid
EEG	Electroencephalogram
EJV	External jugular vein
EMD	Electromechanical dissociation
ERCP	Endoscopic retrograde cholangio-pancreatogram
ERV	Expiratory reserve volume
ESR	Erythrocyte sedimentation rate
ETT	Endo-tracheal tube
FBC	Full blood count
FDP	Fibrin degradation product
FES	Fat embolism syndrome
FEV	Forced expiratory volume
FFP	Fresh frozen plasma
FRC	Functional residual capacity
FVC	Forced vital capacity
GCS	Glasgow coma score
GFR	Glomerular filtration rate
GIT	Gastrointestinal tract
GTN	Glyceryl trinitrate
HDU	High dependency unit
HIV	Human immunodeficiency virus
HPV	Hypoxic pulmonary vasoconstriction
HR	Heart rate
IABP	Intra-aortic balloon pump
IAH	Intra-abdominal hypertension
IAP	Intra-abdominal pressure
ICF	Intracellular fluid
ICP	Intra-cranial pressure
ICU	Intensive care unit
IJV	Internal jugular vein
IL	Interleukin
INR	International normalised ratio
IOP	Intra-optic pressure
IPPV	Intermittent positive pressure ventilation
IRV	Inspiratory reserve volume/Inverse ratio ventilation
ISS	Injury severity scale

ITU	Intensive therapy unit
IVC	Inferior vena cava
JVP	Jugular venous pressure
LD	Lethal dose
LDH	Lactate dehydrogenase
LFT	Liver function test
LMA	Laryngeal mask airway
LOC	Loss of consciousness
LOS	Lower oesophageal sphincter
MAP	Mean arterial pressure
MAWP	Mean airway pressure
MBP	Mean blood pressure
MI	Myocardial infarction
MODS	Multi-organ dysfunction syndrome
MOF	Multi-organ failure
MOFS	Multi-organ failure syndrome
MRI	Magnetic resonance imaging
MV	Minute volume
NO	Nitric oxide
NSAIDs	Non-steroidal anti-inflammatory drugs
ODC	Oxyhaemoglobin dissociation curve
ODP	Operating department practioner
PAF	Platelet activating factor
PAFC	Pulmonary artery floatation catheter
PAH	Para-amino hippuric acid
PAOP	Pulmonary artery occlusion pressure
PAWP	Peak airway pressure
PCA	Patient controlled analgesia
PCV	Pressure controlled ventilation
PE	Pulmonary embolism
PEA	Pulseless electrical activity
PEEP	Positive end expiratory pressure
PEFR	Peak expiratory flow rate
PEG	Percutaneous gastrostomy
PEJ	Percutaneous jejunostomy
PIFR	Peak inspiratory flow rate
PS	Pressure support
PSV	Pressure support ventilation
PT	Prothrombin time
PVR	Pulmonary vascular resistance

RAA	Renin-angiotensin-aldosterone
RBC	Red blood cell
RDS	Respiratory distress syndrome
RQ	Respiratory quotient
RR	Respiratory rate
RTS	Revised trauma score
RV	Residual volume
SBC	Standard bicarbonate
SBE	Standard base excess
SCV	Subclavicular vein
SDH	Subdural haematoma
SIADH	Syndrome of inappropriate antidiuretic hormone
SIMV	Synchronised intermittent mandatory ventilation
SIRS	Systemic inflammatory response syndrome
SV	Stroke volume
SVC	Superior vena cava
SVR	Systemic vascular resistance
TBSA	Total body surface area
TIAE	Tracheo-innominate artery erosion
TIPSS	Transjugular intrahepatic portosystemic shunt
TLC	Total lung capacity
TNF	Tumour necrosis factor
TOE	Transoesophageal echo/echocardiogram/echocardiography
TPN	Total parenteral nutrition/Triphosphopyridine nucleotide
TRALI	Transfusion related acute lung injury
TT	Thrombin time
TTE	Transthoracic echo
U&E	Urea & Electrolytes
VC	Vital capacity
VF	Ventricular fibrillation
VSD	Ventricular septal defect
VT	Ventricular tachycardia
WCC	White cell count

Acknowledgements

We wish to thank our families for their continuing support, and Gavin Smith of Greenwich Medical Media for his patience and encouragement in seeing the book through to press.

Section 1 – MCQs

Q 1. Concerning the post-operative cardiac surgical patient:

A. Ventricular tachycardia (VT) is common

B. Temporary pacing is the treatment of choice for persisting bradyarrhythmias

C. A loop diuretic (e.g. furosemide) is the next line of treatment following an adequate fluid load in a patient with low urine output

D. The incidence of discrete central nervous system (CNS) damage is about 2%

E. Slow recovery of central temperature is suggestive of poor cardiac output (CO)

Q 2. Concerning cardiopulmonary bypass (CPB):

A. The optimal perfusion pressure is 120 mmHg

B. Venous cannulation is normally into the inferior vena cava for closed procedures

C. The arterial cannula is usually inserted in the descending aorta

D. The femoral artery is a recognised site for inserting the arterial cannula

E. The patient is cooled to 25°C if circulatory arrest is necessary

Q 3. The following are commonly seen after coronary artery bypass grafting (CABG):

A. Atrial arrhythmias

B. Basal lung collapse

C. Blood loss of approximately 250 ml in the first hour after surgery

D. New Q waves on electrocardiogram (ECG)

E. Diffuse cerebral injury resulting in an alteration in short term memory

Q 4. Causes of poor cardiac output following cardiac surgery include:

A. Poor myocardial function
B. Cardiac tamponade
C. Bleeding
D. Hypocapnia
E. Alkalosis

Q 5. The following are indicators of poor peripheral perfusion:

A. Hyperthermia
B. Oliguria
C. Confusion
D. Metabolic alkalosis
E. Central cyanosis

Q 6. Heparin:

A. Increases formation of Antithrombin III – Thrombin complex
B. Has a high lipid solubility
C. Is metabolised in the liver
D. May be used in the treatment of disseminated intravascular coagulation (DIC)
E. May lead to hypotension

Q 7. Pulmonary artery catheterisation:

A. Placement can be confirmed by a characteristic waveform
B. Sepsis following catheterisation may lead to endocarditis
C. Is useful in septic shock
D. Wedging of the catheter is necessary in pulmonary infarction
E. Cannot be done via peripheral veins

Q 8. Norepinephrine (noradrenaline):

A. Acts mainly by α-1 adrenoceptors
B. Is excreted in the urine
C. Has a half life of approximately 2 minutes

D. Reduces renal blood flow

E. May increase pulmonary vascular resistance

Q 9. Dopamine:

A. At lower doses (<10 mcg/kg/min) increases contractility and heart rate (HR)

B. Can increase cyclic AMP

C. Has predominantly β-1 effects at higher doses (>10 mcg/kg/min)

D. Is more arrhythmogenic than epinephrine (adrenaline)

E. Vasodilates mesenteric vessels

Q 10. Concerning shock:

A. Pulmonary artery occlusion pressure (PAOP) is usually increased in septic shock

B. Cardiac output is often decreased in hypovolaemic shock

C. Effective management of shock necessitates measurements of both cardiac output and systemic vascular resistance

D. Blood pressure falls in septic shock

E. A urine output of 15 ml/hr is characteristic of class 1 shock

Q 11. Concerning emboli:

A. 80% of systemic arterial emboli originate from the heart

B. 10 ml of gas injected is usually sufficient to cause significant problems

C. Small pulmonary emboli can lead to right heart failure

D. Hypoxia 24 hours after a long bone fracture is likely to be due to pulmonary embolus

E. Aortic thromboemboli usually have an impact in the cerebral arterial system

Q 12. Concerning vascular trauma:

A. Haemodynamic instability is an indication for urgent angiography

B. Contrast computed tomography (CT) is useful for assessing great vessel injury

C. Intimal injuries are the most common vascular injuries

D. Shunting may be necessary for damage control

E. Packing is useful in controlling major arterial bleeds

Q 13. Transfusion:

A. Transfusion related acute lung injury (TRALI) manifests itself classically by severe dyspnoea

B. Graft versus host disease usually occurs within 24 hours

C. Management of WBC mediated transfusion reactions include the immediate cessation of the transfusion

D. Leucodepletion reduces the risk of febrile reactions

E. Massive transfusion is defined as the transfusion of more than half the blood volume in 24 hours

Q 14. Haemorrhagic shock:

A. In class II shock the systolic BP is low

B. Class III shock is associated with a urine output of approximately 10 ml per hour

C. Pulse pressure is decreased in class I shock

D. Class III shock is a loss of approximately 25% of the blood volume

E. Confusion is indicative of class III shock

Q 15. The following are causes of peri-operative arrhythmias:

A. Hypocapnia

B. Hypoxaemia

C. Pain

D. Myocardial infarction (MI)

E. Local anaesthetics

Q 16. The following ECG changes are supportive for the diagnosis of post-operative pulmonary embolus:

A. Right bundle branch block

B. T wave inversion in the anterior chest leads

C. Left axis deviation

D. Atrial fibrillation (AF)

E. Right ventricular strain

Q 17. The following haematological parameters would raise the suspicion of DIC:

A. Decreased platelets
B. Increased fibrinogen
C. Prolonged thrombin time
D. Decreased fibrin degradation products (FDP)
E. Profuse bleeding

Q 18. Concerning intravenous fluids in the critically ill:

A. Approximately 20% of infused normal saline (0.9% NaCl) remains intravascular
B. Hartmann's solution (Ringer's lactate) contains approximately 20 mmol/l potassium
C. Normal saline has a pH of 7.4
D. Hartmann's solution is isotonic
E. Approximately 30% of infused 5% dextrose remains intravascular

Q 19. Concerning the post-operative cardiac surgical patient:

A. VT is common
B. Temporary pacing is generally the treatment of choice for persisting bradyarrhythmias
C. A loop diuretic (e.g. Furosemide) is the second line of treatment, after ensuring adequate fluid load, for low urine output
D. The incidence of discrete CNS damage is approximately 2%
E. Slow recovery of central temperature is suggestive of poor cardiac output

Q 20. The following are commonly seen after CABG:

A. Atrial arrhythmias
B. Basal lung collapse
C. Blood loss of 250 ml in the first post-operative hour
D. New Q waves on ECG
E. Diffuse cerebral injury leading to short term memory alteration

Q 21. Causes of poor cardiac output following cardiac surgery include:

   A. Poor myocardial function
   B. Cardiac tamponade
   C. Bleeding
   D. Hypocapnia
   E. Alkalosis

Q 22. Insertion of a pulmonary artery floatation catheter (PAFC) enables the following:

   A. Measurement of right side cardiac filling pressure
   B. Measurement of left side cardiac filling pressure
   C. Measurement of pulmonary artery pressure
   D. Measurement of cardiac output
   E. Measurement of core blood temperature

Q 23. The following may cause pulseless electrical activity (PEA):

   A. Hypokalaemia
   B. Hypocalcaemia
   C. Open pneumothorax
   D. Cardiac rupture
   E. β-blockers

Q 24. Dopamine:

   A. Stimulates cardiac β-1 receptors
   B. Has a most common complication of tachycardia
   C. When it extravasates causes profound tissue damage
   D. In low doses reduces serum prolactin
   E. May worsen mesenteric perfusion at low doses

Q 25. In septic shock:

   A. Treatment should be with fluid therapy initially
   B. Pulmonary artery floatation catheter is contra-indicated
   C. Vasoactive agents can be useful

D. Norepinephrine does not improve renal function
E. 10% of patients present with myocardial dysfunction

Q 26. Cardiac output:

A. Is the volume of blood ejected from the left ventricle per minute
B. Is proportional to stroke volume (SV)
C. Is inversely related to heart rate
D. Decreases as the filling pressure (preload) increases
E. Decreases as the systemic vascular resistance (afterload) increases

Q 27. The following statements regarding the circulation are correct:

A. The total blood volume is about 5 litres
B. Only about 50% of the intravascular volume is distributed in the systemic arterial circulation
C. Blood pressure = cardiac output × total peripheral resistance
D. In the normal heart, the blood volume is the main determinant of central venous pressure (CVP)
E. A drop in blood pressure results in a reflex increase in heart rate and vasoconstriction mediated by baroceptors in the aorta and carotid sinus

Q 28. Preload (filling pressure):

A. Is dependent upon volume status
B. Is reduced by venodilators
C. Is reduced by diuretics
D. Of the right heart can be measured by the CVP
E. Of the left heart can be measured by the PAOP

Q 29. Afterload:

A. Is the myocardial wall tension developed during systole
B. Is inversely proportional to peripheral vascular resistance
C. Reduction decreases myocardial oxygen requirements
D. Reduction can increase the stroke volume
E. Reduction may increase coronary blood flow

Q 30. Tissue oxygen delivery increases with:

   A. Cardiac output
   B. Haemoglobin concentration
   C. Haemoglobin saturation
   D. Acidosis
   E. Pyrexia

Q 31. Myocardial contractility is reduced by:

   A. Epinephrine (adrenaline)
   B. Hypoxia
   C. Dobutamine
   D. Nitrates
   E. β-blockers

Q 32. Physiological responses to heart failure include:

   A. An increase in heart rate due to activation of the parasympathetic nervous system
   B. Activation of the renin-angiotensin-aldosterone (RAA) system
   C. Increased erythropoietin secretion
   D. Peripheral vasodilatation
   E. Increased sodium and water excretion

Q 33. Cardiac failure:

   A. May be defined as the failure of the heart to meet the metabolic demands of the body at normal filling pressures
   B. Is initially partially compensated through increased myocardial muscle pre-stretching and myocardial contractility (Starling's law)
   C. Is most commonly caused by ischaemic heart disease in Western societies
   D. Is usually associated with a low systemic vascular resistance
   E. Is usually associated with a low PAOP

Q 34. The CVP is typically elevated in:

   A. Hypovolaemia
   B. Congestive cardiac failure

C. The first 6 hours after a general anaesthetic

D. Sepsis

E. Cardiac tamponade

Q 35. CVP monitoring:

    A. Allows assessment of the preload/filling pressure of the left heart

    B. Carries a higher risk of pneumothorax by the subclavian compared with the internal jugular approach

    C. Carries a higher risk of haemothorax by the subclavian compared with the internal jugular approach

    D. Indicates hypovolaemia when the CVP is low

    E. May not reflect the left heart filling pressure in patients with chronic obstructive pulmonary disease (COPD)

Q 36. PAOP:

    A. Is a reflection of left atrial pressure

    B. Is measured by temporary occlusion of a pulmonary vein by a flotation catheter

    C. Must be measured in a cardiac catheter laboratory

    D. Measurement may be complicated by haemoptysis

    E. Measurement may be complicated by pulmonary infarction

Q 37. PAOP:

    A. Can be derived from the CVP and haemoglobin concentration

    B. Measurement involves passage of a pulmonary artery catheter across the interatrial septum

    C. Measurement is appropriate when volume status is uncertain after clinical assessment and measurement of the CVP

    D. Is typically raised in adult respiratory distress syndrome (ARDS)

    E. Is typically raised in septic shock

Q 38. Quantitative measurement of cardiac output can be made using:

    A. CVP and haemoglobin concentration

    B. Thermodilution techniques

C. An oesophageal Doppler probe

D. The Fick principle

E. Mixed venous oxygen saturation and heart rate

Q 39. The following are normal values:

A. CVP: 1–10 mmHg

B. PAOP: 16–28 mmHg

C. Cardiac index: 2.5–4 l/min/m^2

D. Systemic vascular resistance: 350–750 dyn s/cm^5

E. Pulmonary artery pressure: 25/10 mmHg

Q 40. Cardiogenic shock:

A. Is shock due to inability of the heart to maintain the circulation

B. Is characterised by a low cardiac output

C. Is characterised by a low PAOP

D. Is characterised by a low systemic vascular resistance

E. May be caused by papillary muscle rupture

Q 41. Septic shock is characterised by:

A. Increased capillary permeability

B. Vasoconstriction

C. A low cardiac output

D. A high systemic vascular resistance

E. A high capillary artery occlusion pressure

Q 42. On the ECG:

A. The P wave represents ventricular depolarisation

B. The P wave occurs during systole

C. The QRS complex represents ventricular depolarisation

D. The T wave represents ventricular repolarisation

E. Prolongation of the PR interval reflects delayed conduction through the atrioventricular node

Q 43. ST segment depression on the ECG may be caused by:

A. Left ventricular hypertrophy

B. Digoxin therapy

C. Myocardial ischaemia
D. Hyperkalaemia
E. Left bundle branch block

Q 44. MI may be associated with the following ECG features:

A. Left bundle branch block
B. Complete heart block
C. ST segment elevation
D. ST segment depression
E. Normal ECG

Q 45. In post-operative MI:

A. Creatinine kinase MB isoenzyme (CKMB) is the most specific marker of ischaemic myocardial injury
B. Cardiac monitoring is mandatory
C. ST segment elevation indicates the need for immediate administration of thrombolytic therapy
D. Aspirin should be administered
E. Intravenous nitrates improve prognosis

Q 46. Post-myocardial infarction ventricular septal defect (VSD):

A. Causes a diastolic murmur
B. May be confused clinically with mitral regurgitation
C. Causes a left to right shunt
D. Is usually diagnosed by transoesophageal echocardiogram (TOE)
E. Is an indication for insertion of an intra-aortic balloon pump (IABP)

Q 47. The following are consistent with pulmonary embolism (PE):

A. Raised jugular venous pressure (JVP)
B. Type I respiratory failure
C. Normal ECG
D. PEA
E. Dilated right ventricle on ECG

Q 48. Risk of post-operative PE is increased by:

A. Pelvic surgery
B. Anaemia
C. Hip surgery
D. Malignancy
E. Renal failure

Q 49. Post-operative pulmonary oedema:

A. May be non-cardiogenic
B. May be caused by MI in the absence of chest pain
C. Should initially be treated with no more than 24% oxygen to avoid the development of hypercapnia
D. Is appropriately treated with intravenous opiate
E. Is a recognised cause of type I respiratory failure

Q 50. The treatment of acute pulmonary oedema should include:

A. 24% oxygen
B. β-blockers
C. Intravenous diuretic
D. Intravenous nitrate
E. Angiotensin converting enzyme (ACE) inhibitors

Q 51. Hypotension in the post-operative patient may be caused by:

A. Hypovolaemia
B. Hyperkalaemia
C. PE
D. Urinary retention
E. Sepsis

Q 52. Hypotension after cardiac surgery may be caused by:

A. Cardiac tamponade
B. Left ventricular dysfunction
C. Complete heart block
D. Hypovolaemia
E. Systemic inflammatory response syndrome (SIRS)

Q 53. AF after cardiac surgery:

    A. Occurs in 20–40% patients

    B. Is more common in older patients

    C. Is characterised by regular P wave activity but irregular QRS complexes on the ECG

    D. Is usually persistent until electrical or chemical cardioversion is performed

    E. Usually indicates the occurrence of peri-operative MI

Q 54. The treatment of post-operative AF may include:

    A. Correction of electrolyte imbalance

    B. Ventricular rate control with digoxin

    C. Pharmacological cardioversion with amiodarone

    D. Synchronised direct current (DC) cardioversion

    E. Anticoagulation

Q 55. Early complications of aortic valve replacement include:

    A. Complete heart block

    B. Endocarditis

    C. SIRS

    D. Cardiac tamponade

    E. Neurocognitive impairment

Q 56. Signs of cardiac tamponade after cardiac surgery include:

    A. Hypertension

    B. Raised CVP

    C. Kussmaul's sign

    D. Corrigan's sign

    E. Pulsus alternans

Q 57. Pericardiocentesis:

    A. Is only indicated for cardiac tamponade

    B. Is contra-indicated by malignant disease

    C. Is most commonly performed by an apical approach

    D. May be complicated by coronary artery laceration

    E. May be complicated by laceration of the right ventricle

Q 58. Aortic root abscess:

A. May cause complete heart block
B. May cause first degree heart block
C. May cause persistent pyrexia despite appropriate antibiotic therapy
D. Is a contra-indication to aortic valve replacement
E. Is usually diagnosed by transthoracic echo

Q 59. Indications for surgery in endocarditis include:

A. Haemodynamic compromise due to valve dysfunction
B. Penicillin allergy
C. Failure to eradicate infection despite appropriate antibiotic therapy
D. Recurrent thromboembolic events
E. Uncomplicated native valve endocarditis without haemodynamic compromise

Q 60. Aortic dissection:

A. Is predisposed by an inherent weakness of the aortic wall adventitia
B. Is associated with Marfan's syndrome
C. Is associated with hypertension
D. Is associated with pregnancy
E. Is classified as Stanford type B when the ascending aorta is involved

Q 61. Aortic dissection:

A. May cause mitral regurgitation
B. May cause renal failure
C. May cause inferior MI
D. May cause pleural but not pericardial effusion
E. May cause acute lower limb ischaemia

Q 62. In aortic dissection:

A. Magnetic resonance imaging (MRI) is the investigation of choice for unstable patients
B. Echocardiography is able to assess aortic root size, presence of aortic regurgitation and pericardial effusion

C. Intravenous labetalol is appropriate antihypertensive therapy
D. Distal dissections should generally be managed surgically
E. Surgical treatment is contra-indicated when the ascending aorta is involved

Q 63. TOE:

A. Is contra-indicated in the intubated patient
B. Requires monitoring of patient oxygen saturation and heart rhythm
C. Has a sensitivity and specificity of about 95% for the diagnosis of aortic dissection
D. Can be used intraoperatively to monitor left ventricular function
E. Is indicated to assess the intra-operative results of mitral valve repair

Q 64. Dobutamine:

A. Is a positive inotrope
B. Stimulates β-1, β-2, and α-1 receptors
C. Causes vasodilatation and a decrease in peripheral vascular resistance
D. Is indicated in the treatment of cardiogenic shock
E. Results in a lower increase in myocardial oxygen requirements than other inotropes

Q 65. Epinephrine (adrenaline):

A. Stimulates both α- and β-adrenoceptors
B. Causes vasodilatation and a decrease in afterload
C. Reduces myocardial oxygen demand
D. Increases coronary and cerebral perfusion during cardiopulmonary resuscitation
E. Can be given via an endotracheal tube during a cardiac arrest

Q 66. The following statements are correct:

A. Norepinephrine (noradrenaline) predominantly stimulates β-adrenoceptors
B. Norepinephrine is a potent vasoconstrictor

C. Norepinephrine is indicated in the treatment of shock associated with a low peripheral vascular resistance

D. Dopamine is the precursor of epinephrine and norepinephrine

E. Dopamine independently improves outcome in acute renal failure

Q 67. IABP:

A. Should be positioned with the tip of the balloon proximal to the left subclavian artery

B. Is timed to inflate during systole

C. Increases coronary perfusion pressure

D. Increases afterload

E. Requires anticoagulation

Q 68. IABP:

A. Is indicated in acute mitral regurgitation due to papillary muscle rupture

B. Is indicated in acute severe aortic regurgitation

C. Is indicated in aortic dissection

D. May be complicated by lower limb ischaemia

E. May be complicated by pericardial effusion

Q 69. In out-of-hospital suspected cardiac arrest:

A. The first consideration is minimising risk to rescuer and victim

B. The airway should be opened by 'head tilt/chin lift'

C. The victim's breathing should be assessed for 30 seconds before initiating rescue breathing

D. The unconscious self-ventilating victim should be placed in the recovery position

E. Chest compression should be initiated if there are no signs of a circulation after a 10 second assessment

Q 70. In basic life support (BLS):

A. A ratio of 15 chest compressions to two rescue breaths should be used

B. Chest compressions achieve about 50% normal cardiac output

C. Chest compressions should be performed at a rate of 70 per minute
D. Chest compression should depress the sternum by 10 cm
E. Chest compressions should be interrupted for each rescue breath

Q 71. In pulseless ventricular tachycardia/ventricular fibrillation (VT/VF):

A. BLS carries a 20% chance of restoring an effective cardiac rhythm
B. A praecordial thump may restore a cardiac output
C. The chance of successful defibrillation decreases by 10% per minute
D. The recommended energy sequence for the first three successive defibrillations is 200 J, 300 J, 360 J
E. Lidocaine (lignocaine) is the antiarrhythmic drug of choice for shock-resistant VT/VF

Q 72. In cardiac arrest:

A. Cerebral hypoxic injury begins within 3 minutes
B. Drug delivery is optimally achieved via a central vein
C. Epinephrine (adrenaline) 1 mg should be administered every minute during cardiopulmonary resuscitation
D. Open chest cardiac massage is indicated after recent cardiothoracic surgery
E. Associated with trauma, the cervical spine should be protected during airway manipulation

Q 73. In cardiac arrest, drugs that can be administered down the endotracheal tube include:

A. Amiodarone
B. Sodium bicarbonate
C. Atropine
D. Calcium gluconate
E. Lidocaine (lignocaine)

Q 74. PEA:

    A. Is characterised by cardiac arrest with an ECG rhythm other than VT compatible with a cardiac output

    B. May be caused by tension pneumothorax

    C. May be caused by hypovolaemia

    D. Should be treated with 3 mg atropine irrespective of heart rate

    E. Should be treated with epinephrine (adrenaline) 1 mg every 3 minutes of cardiopulmonary resuscitation

Q 1. Positive end expiratory pressure (PEEP):

A. Increases functional residual capacity (FRC)
B. Decreases lung compliance
C. Increases intra-cranial pressure
D. Increases lung barotrauma
E. May increase cardiac output (CO)

Q 2. The following are indicators of failure of mask oxygen therapy at high F_IO_2:

A. Respiratory rate (RR) > 30 breaths per minute
B. Oxygen saturation < 90%
C. PaO_2 < 8 kPa
D. $PaCO_2$ < 7 kPa
E. Dyspnoea

Q 3. Hyponatraemia may be due to:

A. Hypovolaemia
B. Oedema
C. Renal failure
D. Syndrome of inappropriate antidiuretic hormone (SIADH)
E. Diuretics

Q 4. The following are clinical manifestations of barotrauma:

A. Pneumothorax
B. Pneumomediastinum
C. Subcutaneous emphysema
D. Pneumoperitoneum
E. Air embolus

Q 5. **The following may cause respiratory alkalosis:**

   A. Hypothyroidism

   B. Fever

   C. Pain

   D. Anaemia

   E. Pregnancy

Q 6. **Adult respiratory distress syndrome (ARDS):**

   A. Is characterised by pulmonary oedema in the presence of a raised pulmonary artery occlusion pressure (PAOP)

   B. May be caused by acute pancreatitis

   C. May be caused by septicaemia

   D. May complicate cardio-pulmonary bypass

   E. Is managed with steroids, which improve prognosis

Q 7. **Post-operative respiratory failure may be caused by:**

   A. ARDS

   B. Aspiration pneumonia

   C. Basal atelectasis

   D. Opiate analgesia

   E. Pulmonary embolism

Q 8. **Central chemoreceptors:**

   A. Detect the level of O_2 and CO_2 in blood

   B. Are directly stimulated by CO_2

   C. Buffering capacity in cerebrospinal fluid (CSF) is good

   D. CO_2 diffuses slowly between CSF + blood

   E. Normal control of ventilation is mediated by CO_2 homeostasis

Q 9. **Control of ventilation:**

   A. Peripheral chemoreceptors are sensitive to O_2 and are located in the carotid and aortic sinus

   B. Output from peripheral chemoreceptors start to increase at PaO_2 13.3 kPa and stop below PaO_2 4.4 kPa

   C. Concomitant increase in CO_2 potentiates the effect of hypoxia but the response is linear above 5.3 kPa

D. Central chemoreceptors are situated on the dorsal medulla oblongate and thalamus
E. The Hering-Breuer reflex is concerned with lung inflation, the impulses for which are carried within the vagus nerve

Q 10. The following statements refer to lung volumes:

A. Total lung capacity is the maximal volume of air that can be expired following a maximal inspiration
B. Tidal volume is 8–12 ml/kg in adults
C. Expiratory reserve volume is the maximal volume of air that can be expelled after tidal expiration, and is usually over 3000 ml
D. Closing capacity is the lung volume where small air way begin to collapse on inspiration
E. In fit adults at altitude total lung capacity and vital capacity are equal

Q 11. FRC:

A. Is the volume of air remaining in the lungs after a maximal expiration
B. Is usually greater than inspiratory reserve volume
C. When less than closing capacity results in hypoxaemia during tidal ventilation
D. Is increased by continuous positive airways pressure (CPAP)
E. Is increased by regional anaesthesia

Q 12. Compliance:

A. Is the rate of change of gas flow per unit change in pressure $\Delta f/\Delta p$
B. Is a measurement of lung distensibility
C. Is increased in the newborn
D. Is decreased in restrictive lung disease
E. Is increased at low lung volumes

Q 13. Ventilation and perfusion:

A. During spontaneous respiration the majority of inspired gas is directed to the upper parts of the lung
B. Upper parts of the lung are on a steeper part of the compliance curve in spontaneously breathing patients

C. Blood flow is greatest at the base of the lung due to the effects of hydrostatic pressure

D. Altering the mode of ventilation from spontaneous to mechanical has minimal effect on ventilation perfusion ratio in the supine subject

E. Hypoxic pulmonary vasoconstriction (HPV) is a method whereby the lungs decrease the blood supply to the lungs

Q 14. Ventilation and perfusion:

A. Shunt refers to areas of the lung which are well ventilated but with poor blood supply

B. Dead space refers to areas of the lung which are well perfused but poorly ventilated

C. Patients with hypoxaemia due to shunt will benefit from 100% O_2 delivered via a facemask to increase haemoglobin saturation

D. Physiological shunt accounts for about 2% of CO

E. Upper areas of the lung tend towards shunt rather than dead space during mechanical ventilation

Q 15. Pulmonary function tests:

A. FEV_1/FVC ratio is usually of the order of 0.6

B. FEV_1/FVC ratios are more helpful in demonstrating obstructive rather than restrictive lung pathologies

C. In restrictive conditions FEV_1 and FVC are both reduced but the ratio is often increased

D. In obstructive conditions FEV_1 remains constant but the FVC is often increased

E. FVC and FEV_1 are usually measured at the bedside with a peak flow meter

Q 16. Arterial blood gases (ABG):

A. $PaCO_2$ of 4.6 kPa is within the normal range

B. pH is directly proportional to the H^+ content of blood

C. Standard bicarbonate (SBC) is a direct measurement of plasma bicarbonate

D. Decreasing the temperature of a sample decreases the H^+ content

E. Decreasing the temperature of a sample decreases the O_2 content

Q 17. Acid-base homeostasis:

A. The cells of the human body can function over a wide-range of pH values
B. An open buffer system is one in which there is an inexhaustible supply of components
C. Haemoglobin is a more effective buffer in the oxygenate HbO form
D. Haemoglobin and plasma proteins account for nearly half the body's buffering capacity
E. Fully compensated acidosis may result in a pH value of 7.46

Q 18. Metabolic Acidosis:

A. Can be due to intestinal fistulae
B. Is often the result of acid ingestion (iatrogenic)
C. Patients should be given sodium bicarbonate to correct any deficit
D. May be compounded by hyperventilation
E. May result from salicylate ingestion

Q 19. pH 7.1, PCO_2 2.8 kPa, PO_2 13 kPa, HCO_3^- 7 mmol/l, SBC 8 mmol/l, actual base excess (ABE) − 21 mmol/l, standard base excess (SBE) − 20 mmol/l, Glucose 22 mmol/l. Which of the following are true for this patient:

A. $NaHCO_3$ 8.4% 100 ml should be given as soon as possible
B. The primary problem is due to loss of HCO_3^- from the body
C. Controlling blood sugar is a primary concern and should be the first priority
D. The patient may require 10 litres of intravenous fluid
E. This patient may be oliguric

Q 20. pH 7.56, PCO_2 7.2 kPa, PO_2 9 kPa, HCO_3^- 45 mmol/l, SBC 35 mmol/l, ABE 10 mmol/l, SBE 6 mmol/l, Sat 90%. Which of the following are true for this patient:

A. This patient may be taking diuretics
B. Hypoxia may be secondary
C. Treatment options include normal saline infusion
D. The urine pH will be about 6
E. They may have Conn's syndrome

Q 21. **Respiratory acidosis:**

  A. Caused by asthma is usually self limiting
  B. Is not of primary concern in multi-trauma victims who may have many other injuries
  C. Normal pH may be achieved safely with small amounts of sodium bicarbonate
  D. Despite compensation a patient with pH 7.38 may still have a $PaCO_2$ of 8 kPa
  E. The bicarbonate buffer system is not useful since the mechanism for CO_2 removal may be impaired

Q 22. **Respiratory alkalosis:**

  A. When caused by salicylate poisoning is associated with metabolic acidosis
  B. Occurs with pneumonia
  C. Oxygen therapy should be avoided initially until the diagnosis of cause is made
  D. When occurring in patients with deep vein thrombosis (DVT) is usually clinically irrelevant
  E. May result in the patient passing urine of pH 5.5

Q 23. **Regarding oxygen delivery:**

  A. Is more efficient at Hb 10 g/dl than 15 g/dl
  B. Is decreased at altitude due to reduced CO
  C. Increasing the inspired oxygen concentration to 50% increases the oxygen content of blood by 50%
  D. A patient with Hb 10 g/dl breathing air will have greater oxygen delivery than a patient with Hb 8 g/dl breathing 50% O_2
  E. The dissolved fraction of O_2 contributes upto 10% of the total oxygen carrying capacity

Q 24. **Hypoxia:**

  A. Carbon monoxide poisoning causes histotoxic hypoxia
  B. Stagnant hypoxia responds well to oxygen therapy
  C. Altitude results in anaemic hypoxia
  D. Stagnant hypoxia leads to low venous oxygen content
  E. Cyanotic heart disease is a cause of hypoxic hypoxia

Q 25. Oxygen therapy:

A. Stops shivering in post-operative patients by reducing the metabolic demand for oxygen
B. The oxygen concentration delivered by the Hudson mask may be accurately derived from the fresh gas flow
C. At higher peak inspiratory flow rates (PIFR) the oxygen concentration is increased because more air is entrained
D. The maximal oxygen concentration that can be delivered by nasal specs is 40%
E. 10 l/min via the Hudson mask gives an oxygen concentration of over 80%

Q 26. Oxygen therapy:

A. Venturi masks are examples of fixed performance oxygen delivery systems
B. Oxygen concentration is independent of peak inspiratory flow rate (PIFR) but not minute volume
C. Red masks deliver 40% oxygen at 10 l/min
D. Is less useful than Hudson mask in COPD patients since they tend to deliver higher concentrations of oxygen
E. Require more oxygen flow (l/min) to reach the same oxygen concentration than the equivalent Hudson mask

Q 27. Respiratory failure:

A. Type I there is $\downarrow$ PaO_2 and $\downarrow$ or normal $PaCO_2$
B. Type II there is normal PaO_2 but $\uparrow$ $PaCO_2$
C. Type I may be due to pneumonia
D. Type I is associated with Guillain Barré syndrome
E. Type I is associated with ARDS

Q 28. Respiratory failure:

A. Type II failure is easier to treat than type I
B. Kyphoscoliosis usually produces respiratory failure without elevation in $PaCO_2$
C. Type II failure is not associated with tachypnoea
D. Flail chest results in type I failure since CO_2 is lost to the atmosphere via an open pneumothorax
E. Mechanical obstruction of the airway is associated with type I failure

Q 29. The following are reliable signs of respiratory failure:

A. Cyanosis

B. Lowered level of consciousness

C. Tachypnoea

D. Tachycardia

E. Use of accessory muscles of respiration

Q 30. The following are indications for instituting respiratory support:

A. $PaO_2 < 8\,kPa$ breathing $10\,l/min\ O_2$ via a venturi mask

B. Tidal volume $(V_t) < 5\,ml/kg$

C. Glasgow coma score (GCS) of 10

D. $PaCO_2 > 7\,kPa$

E. Intra-operative tracheostomy formation

Q 31. Intermittent positive pressure ventilation (IPPV):

A. Differs from spontaneous ventilation in that expiration is active

B. Can lead to acid/base disturbances

C. Pneumothoracies should not be drained prior to instituting IPPV since the resulting air leak makes ventilation inefficient

D. May worsen shunt leading to hypoxaemia

E. May cause an initial increase in blood pressure

Q 32. IPPV:

A. Reduces cardiac output (CO)

B. Seldom requires sedation unless the patient is anxious

C. May reduce blood pressure on correction of acidosis

D. Has no effect on the kidney

E. May increase intra-cranial pressure

Q 33. Initiating IPPV:

A. F_iO_2 should be set to 1.0 (100% Oxygen)

B. Tidal volume (V_t) should be 6–8 ml/kg

C. Oxygen is mixed with nitrous oxide to prevent pulmonary atelectasis in the intensive care unit (ICU)

D. The I:E ratio is often extended to 1:3 in asthmatic patients

E. PEEP should be applied as soon as possible

Q 34. Controlled mandatory ventilation (CMV):

- **A.** Minute volume is set on the ventilator
- **B.** RR depends on the patient's inspiratory effort
- **C.** Peak pressure is controlled by the ventilator
- **D.** Is useful for patients with poor respiratory compliance
- **E.** Is not a weaning mode

Q 35. Synchronised intermittent mandatory ventilation (SIMV):

- **A.** Minute volume is not constant
- **B.** May result in spontaneous and mandatory breaths being delivered simultaneously resulting in dangerously high peak airway pressures
- **C.** Muscle relaxation is usually required to minimise increases in peak airway pressure
- **D.** Is a weaning mode
- **E.** Improves perfusion and ventilation matching over controlled mandatory ventilation (CMV)

Q 36. Pressure controlled ventilation (PCV):

- **A.** Is favoured when pulmonary compliance is high
- **B.** Is a weaning mode
- **C.** The square wave pressure trace optimises oxygenation
- **D.** Volume and RR are set on the ventilator
- **E.** Muscle relaxation is usually required

Q 37. Pressure support ventilation (PSV):

- **A.** Requires no sedation
- **B.** Is a weaning mode
- **C.** Muscle relaxation is occasionally required
- **D.** Tidal volume is set on the ventilator
- **E.** RR depends on ventilator and patient initiated breaths

Q 38. The following are mechanisms for optimising lung volume:

- **A.** PEEP is mainly used during spontaneous ventilation
- **B.** CPAP is a weaning mode

C. Both PEEP and CPAP improve haemodynamic stability by increasing diastolic blood pressure

D. Inverse ratio ventilation (IRV) involves active expiration

E. IRV may lead to respiratory acidosis

Q 39. Weaning from mechanical ventilation:

A. Opioids should be discontinued

B. Should not be routinely attempted from PCV

C. Patients should be put onto a T-piece once the SIMV rate has been reduced to 8 breaths per minute

D. Patients should be put onto a T-piece once the PEEP level is $10\,cmH_2O$

E. Once a patient has been put on to T-piece spontaneous ventilation they should not go back onto PSV on a ventilator

Q 40. Endo-tracheal intubation:

A. The correct diameter for a paediatric endo-tracheal tube (ETT) is determined by the formula Age/2 + 12

B. The correct diameter for an adult ETT is 9 mm for males

C. The correct length for an adult ETT is 25 cm for females

D. Sellicks manouvre aims to aid intubation

E. Cricoid pressure should be applied with a force of 40 N

Q 41. Airway:

A. Nasal intubation is less cardio vascularly stimulating than oral because laryngoscopy is not required

B. Nasal intubation is favoured in children

C. Nasal intubation is more uncomfortable and requires more sedation than oral

D. Intubation is mandatory if GCS < 8

E. Tracheostomy is more suitable to ventilate obese patients

Q 42. ARDS:

A. May occur after cardio-pulmonary bypass

B. Is known to be associated with malignant hypertension

C. A high plasma amylase concentration may be seen

D. Is caused by raised intra-cranial pressure

E. Infection is the commonest cause

Q 43. The following criteria must be met to define ARDS:

A. The pulmonary artery wedge pressure must be greater than 18 mmHg

B. There must be bilateral fluffy infiltrates on the chest X-ray (CXR)

C. There must be the need for mechanical ventilation

D. There must be high airway pressures

E. The $PaO_2:F_IO_2$ ratio is >27 kPa

Q 44. ARDS:

A. Has a similar pathophysiology to the systemic inflammatory response syndrome (SIRS)

B. Microvascular obliteration is an initiating event

C. Capillary endothelial damage is central to the pathological process

D. A protein rice exudate fills the alveoli due to large hydrostatic forces

E. A fibrosing-alveolitis type reaction is an early pathological sign in severe cases

Q 45. The management of ARDS:

A. Fluids should be given liberally as there is likely to be co-existing septicaemia or hypoperfusion that requires resuscitation

B. A pulmonary artery flotation catheter should always be inserted

C. Normocapnia should be maintained to avoid acidosis

D. Moderate hypoxaemia (PaO_2 > 8 kPa) should be tolerated

E. Increased peak airway pressure has to be accepted in order to reduce CO_2

Q 46. The management of ARDS:

A. PEEP should not be applied since the airway pressure will already be high

B. Increasing FRC will improve oxygenation

C. IRV increases mean airway pressure (MAWP) without increase in peak airway pressure
D. IRV optimises gas exchange
E. Nitric oxide may be given intravenously to help resistant hypoxia

Q 47. ARDS:

A. Poly trauma associated with ARDS carries a grave prognosis
B. Late deaths from ARDS are often due to the precipitating cause
C. Most survivors are asymptomatic
D. 50% of survivors show signs of lung fibrosis on laboratory testing
E. Pneumothoracies, once drained aid ventilation by reducing the peak airway pressure via the air leak

Q 48. Open pneumothorax:

A. Is less clinically significant than closed pneumothorax since pressure in the lungs equilibrates with atmospheric pressure
B. The lung on the side of a penetrating injury does not contribute to ventilation
C. Air exchange occurs between the collapsed and healthy lung
D. There will be no mediastinal shift since the affected lung is open to the atmosphere
E. There may be bradypnoea to compensate for the air leak

Q 49. Pneumothorax:

A. Closed pneumothorax is relatively common and may not be clinically significant
B. In tension pneumothorax air can only escape via the bronchial tree
C. In tension pneumothorax there may be tracheal deviation towards the collapsed lung
D. There may be an increase of 40 mmHg in intrapleural pressure on the affected side
E. Tension pneumothorax is usually diagnosed by CXR

Q 50. The following concern CO_2 transport in blood:

    A. CO_2 is 20 times more soluble than O_2

    B. CO_2 is transported as HCO_3^-, accounting for upto 50% of carriage in blood

    C. HCO_3^- is mainly buffered by plasma proteins

    D. Carbamino compounds are mainly formed with plasma proteins

    E. 70% of HCO_3^- formed from CO_2 in the red blood cell (RBC) diffuses into the plasma

Q 51. The following relate to the transport of CO_2 in blood:

    A. Plasma proteins are significantly involved in the buffering of H^+ liberated during the transport of CO_2

    B. Deoxyhaemoglobin has less buffering capacity than oxyhaemoglobin because of the lower pH (7.36) of venous blood

    C. The Haldane effect allows for greater uptake of CO_2

    D. Chloride shift refers to the movement of Cl^- out of the RBC to allow inward movement of HCO_3^-

    E. RBC in venous blood has less Cl^- than arterial blood

Q 52. Oxygen transport in blood:

    A. Haemoglobin in a complex carbohydrate of 65,000 Daltons

    B. There are four haem containing subgroups, each being a complex of perphyrin and Fe^{3+}

    C. The oxygen dissociation curve is sigmoid because of the differing affinities of the haem groups to O_2

    D. 1 g Hb can carry 1.38 ml of O_2

    E. Increasing Hb from 12 g/dl to 15 g/dl has little effect in increasing the oxygen carrying capacity unless the PaO_2 is also increased

Q 53. Oxyhaemoglobin dissociation curve (ODC):

    A. Left shift increases the slope of the curve

    B. Right shift increases the affinity of Hb for O_2

    C. The Bohr effect is most prominent in the lungs

D. Increasing temperature reduces the affinity of Hb for O_2
E. 2,3-Diphosphoglycerate (2,3-DPG) generated by RBC glycolysis binds avidly to oxyhaemoglobin

Q 54. ODC:

A. Mixed venous saturation corresponds to P50
B. Methaemoglobin is formed when ferrous iron in Hb is reduced to the ferric form
C. Myoglobin has a non-sigmoid dissociation curve because of its greater affinity for O_2
D. Fetal Hb gives up O_2 more easily than adult Hb, which improves tissue oxygenation at low PaO_2
E. Carbon monoxide dissociation curve is to the left of myoglobin

Q 55. Oxygen toxicity:

A. Is rare if P_iO_2 (partial pressure of inspired oxygen) is less than 60 kPa
B. Hyperoxia increases surfactant levels in a bid to keep the airways open
C. Is usually asymptomatic and painless until loss of consciousness
D. Infants are less susceptible since they cannot increase surfactant levels easily
E. May occur during diving

Q 56. Surface tension in the alveoli:

A. Is defined by Laplace's law
B. The wall tension is inversely proportional to the transmural pressure
C. Gas tends to flow from large radius alveoli to smaller radius alveoli to equilibrate the pressure
D. Surfactant, a phospholipid prevents, airway collapse by increasing surface tension in smaller alveoli
E. Surfactant is produced by type II alveolar cells

Q 57. The following statements refer to dead space:

A. Anatomical dead space is 5 ml/kg

B. Physiological dead space consists of anatomical dead space minus alveolar dead space

C. Alveolar dead space corresponds to those parts of the lung which are ventilated but not perfused

D. Physiological dead space may be measured using Fowler's nitrogen washout method

E. Alveolar dead space may be estimated using the Bohr equation

Q 1. The following are indicators of a severe attack acute pancreatitis:

A. Plasma calcium > 2.6 mmol/l
B. Arterial pO_2 < 8 kPa
C. Amylase > three times upper limit of laboratory norm
D. Blood glucose > 8 mmol/l
E. White cell count (WCC) > 15×10^9/l

Q 2. The following are factors which increase risk of rebleeding following a gastrointestinal haemorrhage:

A. Malignancy
B. Acute rather than chronic ulcer
C. Shock on admission
D. Age < 60 years
E. Gastric ulcer

Q 3. Concerning severe pancreatitis:

A. Hypocalcaemia is the most common metabolic problem
B. Coagulopathy is usually the first organ system failure to manifest itself
C. Failure of two organ systems is associated with 90% mortality
D. Solid, infected pancreatic necrosis will often respond to intravenous antibiotics
E. Positive end expiratory pressure (PEEP) may be useful in managing respiratory failure

Q 4. Concerning acute renal failure (ARF):

A. Ultrasound should be performed early
B. Supravesical obstruction is common
C. Insertion of a double J stent is the preferred treatment of supravesical obstruction

D. A unilateral dilated collecting duct system requires urgent decompression and subsequent renography

E. For pelvic malignancy causing ARF nephrostomy insertion is the treatment of choice

Q 5. Concerning thoracic trauma:

A. Chest trauma is responsible for approximately 25% of trauma deaths

B. Most patients with chest injuries ultimately require thoracotomy

C. Penetrating chest wounds often require formal surgery utilising cardiopulmonary bypass

D. Massive haemothorax is defined as >750 ml blood in the chest cavity

E. Continuing blood loss of >50 ml/h is an indication for thoracotomy

Q 6. Characteristic injuries of blunt thoracic trauma include:

A. Fractured sternum

B. Transected aorta

C. Pulmonary contusion

D. Ruptured spleen

E. Bilateral rib fractures

Q 7. Causes of hypoxia in thoracic trauma include:

A. Blood loss

B. Cardiac tamponade

C. Pulmonary contusion

D. Ventilatory failure

E. Mediastinal disruption

Q 8. The following drugs require dose alteration in renal failure:

A. Paracetamol

B. Heparin

C. Morphine

D. Ranitidine

E. Metoclopramide

Q 9. Subdural haematoma (SDH):

A. Is associated with a 20% mortality in cases of simple SDH

B. Following decompression, management is aimed at decreasing cerebral swelling

C. Multiple SDH is associated with a mortality as high as 90%

D. Is due to the tearing of bridging vessels

E. Is classically associated with a lucid interval

Q 10. Concerning shock after a spinal injury:

A. Absent reflexes suggest spinal shock

B. Hypotension and tachycardia suggest neurogenic shock

C. Tachycardia and flaccid muscle is common in spinal shock

D. Bradycardia is a feature of spinal shock

E. Vasopressors may be required in neurogenic shock

Q 11. Concerning smoke inhalation injuries:

A. The half life of carboxyhaemoglobin (COHb) breathing 100% oxygen is less than 1 h

B. High flow oxygen should be given until the COHb level is less than 5%

C. Smoke inhalation causes thermal damage to the whole respiratory tract

D. Soot in the mouth is an indication for fibre-optic laryngoscopy

E. Intubation should be avoided

Q 12. Gastrointestinal stress ulceration:

A. Is rare

B. Causes significant bleeds in 5% of cases

C. Has a mortality which is influenced by prophylaxis

D. Can be prevented by the use on H_2 antagonists in all critically ill patients

E. Often necessitates surgical intervention

Q 13. Enteral nutrition is contra-indicated in the following circumstances in the critically ill patient:

A. Small bowel obstruction
B. Inflammatory bowel disease
C. Dysphagia
D. Small bowel fistulae
E. Diarrhoea

Q 14. The following are necessary daily for patients on total parenteral nutrition (TPN):

A. Full blood count (FBC)
B. Albumin
C. Calcium
D. Urea
E. Glucose

Q 15. Concerning clinical evaluation of pelvic injuries:

A. Rectal examination is often unnecessary
B. The patient should have a urethral catheter inserted in all cases to monitor urine output
C. Antero-posterior (AP) compression injuries are usually more severe than lateral compression injuries
D. Pelvic stabilisation is the first priority
E. Unstable pelvic ring fractures are associated with a high mortality

Q 16. Concerning thermal regulation:

A. Hyperthermia is defined as a body temperature above 39°C
B. Respiratory acidosis occurs with hyperthermia
C. Malignant hyperpyrexia is related to the use of volatile anaesthetic agents
D. The nervous system is most often affected in hyperthermia
E. Central lines should be changed at 5 day intervals

Q 17. Anastamotic leakage:

    A. Is uncommon

    B. Has a higher incidence in shocked patients

    C. When suspected merits an early 2nd look procedure

    D. There is no role for CT scanning

    E. Early nutritional support is advisable

Q 18. Concerning the cephalosporins:

    A. Cefuroxime is a 3rd generation cephalosporin

    B. Approximately 25% of patients with penicillin hypersensitivity are also hypersensitive to the cephalosporins

    C. They have variable intestinal absorption

    D. They are generally metabolised in the liver

    E. 3rd generation cephalosporins are less active against gram-positive organisms than 2nd generation

Q 19. The following criteria allow for non-operative management of liver injuries:

    A. Haemodynamically stable patient

    B. Persistent abdominal pain

    C. Blood transfusion requirement of 2 units

    D. Intra-hepatic haematoma on CT scan

    E. Haemoperitoneum <1 l on CT scan

Q 20. The following are indications for laparotomy in abdominal trauma:

    A. Peritonitis

    B. Persistent shock

    C. Evisceration

    D. Uncontrolled haemorrhage

    E. Gunshot wounds

Q 21. The following are recognised post-operative complications following hepato-biliary surgery for trauma:

    A. Rebleeding

    B. Bile leaks usually requiring further surgery

    C. Ischaemic segments

D. Subhepatic sepsis in approximately 20% of cases

E. Infected fluid collections rarely

Q 22. Concerning mortality after liver injury:

A. The overall mortality is approximately 25%

B. Penetrating injury carries a mortality of 15–20%

C. Blunt injury has a lower mortality than penetrating injury

D. Mortality of blunt hepatic injury is approximately 10% if only the liver is injured

E. Bleeding causes the majority of deaths

Q 23. Blunt trauma to the pancreas:

A. May be clinically occult

B. Abdominal radiographs may show retroperitoneal air

C. Endoscopic retrograde cholangio-pancreatogram (ERCP) is the best investigation

D. Serum amylase is a good investigation

E. Duct damage may be missed at laparotomy

Q 24. The following complications are associated with pancreatic trauma:

A. Pseudocyst

B. Pancreatic fistula

C. Ascites

D. Pancreatic abscess

E. Acute pancreatitis

Q 25. The post-operative hepatic transplant patient:

A. Should resume enteral feeding as soon as possible

B. Steroids are usually continued for at least 1 year

C. Liver function tests (LFTs) are performed daily

D. Cyclosporin is often given in combination with azathioprine as immunosuppressive

E. Acute rejection occurs in approximately half the patients

Q 26. The following are contra-indications to liver transplantation:

A. Hepatocellular carcinoma

B. Extrahepatic malignancy

C. Systemic sepsis

D. Liver metastases from sarcomata

E. Cardiopulmonary disease

Q 27. Acute renal failure:

A. Carries a mortality of approximately 10%

B. Oliguria in an adult is defined as a urine output less than 400 ml per day

C. Mortality increases to 70% if one other organ system is involved

D. Sequelae include hypercalcaemia and hypokalaemia

E. May lead to pericarditis

Q 28. The following may cause post-operative hepatic dysfunction:

A. Sepsis

B. Pancreatitis

C. Transfusion

D. Hypoxia

E. Surgery

Q 29. The following are major inflammatory mediators in systemic inflammatory response syndrome (SIRS):

A. Platelet activating factor (PAF)

B. Tumour necrosis factor (TNF) β

C. Interleukin 1

D. Interleukin 8

E. Interleukin 5

Q 30. The following endocrine responses occur after major trauma:

A. Increased prolactin

B. Decreased anti-diuretic hormone (ADH)

C. Increased thyroxine

D. Increased catecholamines

E. Increased cortisol

Q 31. **In patients with renal failure, dose modification may be necessary with the following antibiotics:**

A. Ampicillin
B. Cefuroxime
C. Benzyl penicillin
D. Gentamicin
E. Metronidazole

Q 32. **Regarding head injury:**

A. The mortality associated with an acute subdural haematoma is approximately double that of acute epidural haematoma
B. Skull fracture is associated with a 20-fold increase in incidence of extradural haematoma
C. Patients with acute subdural haematoma may have a lucid interval
D. Rapid deceleration injuries are associated with subdural haematoma
E. Contrecoup injuries are often more serious than coup injuries

Q 33. **The following are radiological signs of major thoracic trauma:**

A. Mediastinal widening
B. Fractured 2nd rib
C. Fractured sternum
D. Mediastinal emphysema
E. Loss of aortic definition

Q 34. **Concerning enteral nutrition in the ICU patient:**

A. Where intra-cranial pressure (ICP) is elevated sodium restricted feeds are appropriate
B. High volume energy dense feeds are used for patients with severe burns
C. Glutamine supplementation is essential to prevent skeletal muscle catabolism
D. A typical 2000 ml feed would provide approximately 35 g protein
E. 100 ml of standard polymeric enteral feed provides approximately 100 kcal energy

Q 35. The following are complications of enteral nutrition:

  A. Aspiration
  B. Hypoglycaemia
  C. Hypercapnia
  D. Fluid overload
  E. Infection

Q 36. Concerning ballistic thoracic injuries:

  A. Witnessed cardiac arrest is an indication for resuscitative thoracotomy
  B. Pneumothorax is the commonest injury
  C. 80% of patients with a haemothorax can be treated with tube thoracostomy alone
  D. Pericardiocentesis is of limited value
  E. Exploratory thoracotomy is the treatment of choice for transmediastinal injuries

Q 37. Concerning head injuries:

  A. Epidural haematoma classically present with a lucid interval
  B. Acute SDH have a better prognosis than epidural haematoma
  C. Maintenance of cerebral perfusion pressure (CPP) is essential in their management
  D. ICP is normally 15–25 mmHg in an adult
  E. CPP should be maintained above 60 mmHg

Q 38. Treatment of raised ICP includes:

  A. CSF drainage
  B. Prophylactic hyperventilation
  C. Intravenous 20% mannitol
  D. Sedation
  E. Hypothermia

Q 39. The following monitoring is necessary in cases of acute cervical spinal cord injury:

  A. Arterial blood pressure
  B. Pulmonary artery occlusion pressure
  C. End-tidal CO_2

D. Pulse oximetry

E. Urinary output

Q 40. Burns:

A. Mortality associated with a concomitant inhalation injury is 30% greater than that without inhalate injury

B. Inhalation injury commonly results in hypoxaemia associated with bronchospasm and bronchorrhoea

C. Burn wound sepsis is the leading cause of death

D. The hypermetabolic response to burn injury peaks at 48 h

E. Burns patients suffer a marked protein catabolism

Q 41. The following are indications for surgery in acute pancreatitis:

A. Positive fine needle aspirate

B. Sepsis

C. Peritonitis

D. Failure to respond to ICU therapy

E. Respiratory insufficiency

Q 42. The following are suggestive of pre-renal renal failure:

A. Urine sodium < 20 mmol/l

B. Urine osmolality > 500 mosm/kg H_2O

C. Fractional excretion of sodium $> 1\%$

D. Urine creatinine/plasma creatinine < 20

E. Muddy brown granular casts

Q 43. Fluid balance:

A. A 70 kg man has approximately 28 l fluid in the interstitial compartment

B. Approximately 95% potassium is extracellular

C. The daily requirement of sodium is 1–2 mmol/kg/day

D. Hartmann's solution is preferred to normal saline in patients with renal failure

E. The stress response to surgery leads to sodium retention

Q 44. Fat embolism:

A. Leads to the fat embolism syndrome (FES) in 20% of cases
B. Is frequently seen in patients with acute pancreatitis
C. Occurs in association with reaming of long bones
D. Necessitates heparinisation
E. Requires management by ventilation

Q 45. Characteristics of the FES include:

A. Pulmonary insufficiency
B. Thrombocytosis
C. Conjunctival haemorrhages
D. Petechial rash
E. Cerebral signs

Q 46. Causes of hypoxia in thoracic trauma include:

A. Blood loss
B. Tamponade
C. Pulmonary contusion
D. Ventilatory failure
E. Mediastinal disruption

Q 47. Clearance of the following drugs is reduced in ICU patients with hepatic dysfunction:

A. Midazolam
B. Fentanyl
C. Diazepam
D. Thiopentone
E. Furosemide (frusemide)

Q 48. The following are risk factors for the development of acute tubular necrosis (ATN):

A. Diabetes mellitus
B. Infection
C. Malnutrition
D. Hypovolaemia
E. Increasing age

Q 49. The following drugs may cause ARF:

- **A.** Cephalosporins
- **B.** Morphine
- **C.** Dextran
- **D.** Cotrimoxazole
- **E.** Benzyl penicillin

Q 50. The following would be indications to transfer a patient to a burns centre:

- **A.** Chemical burns
- **B.** 15% 2nd degree burns in a patient aged 60
- **C.** 10% burns in an 8 year old boy
- **D.** An electrical burn with an entry wound on the finger and the patient unable to flex the finger
- **E.** 10% 3rd degree burns to the chest in a 25 year old

Q 51. Lactic acidosis:

- **A.** Is characterised by a normal anion gap
- **B.** Is most commonly caused by poor tissue perfusion
- **C.** May be caused by metformin
- **D.** Impairs myocardial contractility
- **E.** Should usually be treated by the administration of sodium bicarbonate

Q 52. Disseminated intravascular coagulation (DIC) is characterised by:

- **A.** Increased fibrinogen concentration
- **B.** Increased fibrinogen degradation products
- **C.** Prolonged activated partial thromboplastin time (APTT)
- **D.** Thrombocythaemia
- **E.** Fragmented red cells on blood film

Q 53. DIC may be caused by:

- **A.** Gram-negative septicaemia
- **B.** Myocardial infarction
- **C.** Burns

D. Pulmonary embolism

E. Haemolytic blood transfusion reactions

Q 54. pH 7.27, pCO$_2$ 3.7 kPa, pO$_2$ 12.6 kPa, HCO$_3$ 14 mmol/l, base excess – 10 mmol/l (on air). These arterial blood gases are characteristic of:

A. Respiratory acidosis

B. Respiratory failure

C. Acute renal failure

D. Septic shock

E. Lactic acidosis type A

Q 55. pH 7.27, pCO$_2$ 7.9 kPa, pO$_2$ 7.1 kPa, HCO$_3$ 24 mmol/l, base excess 2 mmol/l (on air). These arterial blood gases are characteristic of:

A. Type I respiratory failure

B. Chronic CO$_2$ retention

C. Opiate toxicity

D. Acute life-threatening asthma

E. Benzodiazepine overdose

Q 56. SIRS:

A. May be precipitated by tumour invasion

B. May result from acute hypoxaemia post-operatively

C. Is less likely in burns victims since they have a reduced immune response

D. Is due primarily to an abnormal immune reaction

E. Usually results in multi-organ dysfunction syndrome (MODS)

Q 57. SIRS may be diagnosed by:

A. Peripheral temperature $> 38.5°C$

B. Core temperature of 35.8°C

C. Tachycardia of 95 beats per minute

D. Respiratory alkalosis with a PaCO$_2$ of 4.2 kPa

E. WCC of 3.9 x 10^9/l (with 11% neutrophils)

Q 58. SIRS:

  A. Can occur without active injection
  B. Results in cool peripheries due to systolic hypotension
  C. Can result in respiratory acidosis due to hypoperfusion
  D. The patient may have deranged clotting due to liver hypoperfusion
  E. Hypotension is exaccerbated by nitric oxide mediated vasodilatation

Q 59. Multi-organ dysfunction syndrome:

  A. Is a direct effect of end-organ inflammation
  B. Oliguria is a late sign suggesting that organ failure has occurred
  C. Gut hypoperfusion and mucosal atrophy is proposed to have a role in propagating the inflammatory reaction
  D. Is usually irreversible
  E. In the lungs results in ARDS

Q 60. Management of MODS:

  A. Fluid therapy should be used sparingly since tissue oedema and hypoperfusion may be worsened
  B. Inotropes which increase afterload are avoided since they can deteriorate myocardial function
  C. There is no place for β agonists since they exacerbate peripheral vasodilatation
  D. Invasive measurement of cardiac output is mandatory to guide treatment
  E. Arterial cannulation is avoided because of the risk of distal ischaemia

Q 61. Prognosis in MOF:

  A. Is improved in burns patients because they are treated in specialist centres
  B. Mortality rate is 95% on 4th day with three organs failed
  C. Mortality rate is 20% on 1st day with two organs failed
  D. Is worse at the extremes of age
  E. Is improved in sepsis since the infecting precipitant may be isolated, cultured and treated

Q 62. Electrolyte composition:

    A. Intracellular K^+ concentration is normally $>150\,mmol/l$

    B. Ca^{2+} is almost entirely extracellular

    C. The daily requirement of Ca^{2+} is $1\,mmol/kg/day$

    D. Mg^{2+} is mainly extracellular

    E. Extracellular HCO_3^- is three times as concentrated as intracellular

Q 63. The following statements concern crystalloid solutions:

    A. 5% dextrose has a similar osmolality to blood

    B. Hartmann's solution has equal concentrations of Na^+ and Cl^-

    C. Dextrose saline is distributed equally in intracellular fluid (ICF) and extracellular fluid (ECF)

    D. N/saline is hypertonic to blood

    E. Hartmann's solution is isotonic to blood

Q 64. The following are appropriate replacement therapies for the fluid loss:

    A. Peritonitis and fresh frozen plasma (FFP)

    B. Vomiting and D/saline

    C. Diabetes mellitus and Hartmann's solution

    D. Diabetes insipidus and 5% dextrose

    E. Burns and blood

Q 65. Nutrition:

    A. Body mass index (BMI) is $weight^2/height$

    B. Normal BMI is 22–28

    C. Nitrogen requirement is usually $9\,g/day$ for an adult male

    D. Energy requirements are $10–20\,kcal/kg$ for adult females per day

    E. In catabolic patients 1g nitrogen should be given for every $80–100\,kcal$ energy

Q 66. Nutrition in organ failure – the following are appropriate:

    A. Respiratory disease – low carbohydrate, high fat

    B. Renal failure – low nitrogen, high fat

C. Cardiac impairment – low sodium, high volume

D. Liver disease – low nitrogen, low carbohydrate

E. Cerebral impairment – low glucose

Q 67. Nutrition – routes of feeding:

A. The parenteral route is favoured during acute phases of illness on ICU since fluid balance is better controlled

B. Enteral feeding often requires the use of mucosal protection such as sucralfate, since it is directly irritant to the gastric lining

C. Enteral feeding increases the risk of nosocomial pneumonia

D. Hyperglycaemia is only associated with parenteral nutrition in diabetic patients

E. Bowel sounds are a good predictor of gut function

Q 68. Nutrition – physiology:

A. Fats and carbohydrates are completely oxidised to CO_2 and water in the body

B. Protein usually makes up less than 20% of dietary intake

C. A high protein diet increases metabolic rate

D. Respiratory quotient (RQ) for fat is higher than carbohydrate

E. Protein consumption has a significant effect on the overall RQ value

Q 1. **Concerning brainstem death (BSD):**

  A. Electroencephalogram (EEG) recording is necessary in the UK to confirm BSD

  B. 24 hours must elapse between the first and second set of brainstem tests

  C. The vestibulo-ocular reflex is tested by injecting 5 ml of ice-cold water into each external auditory meatus

  D. Apnoea is tested for by disconnecting from the ventilator and insufflating with 6 l/min oxygen until $PaCO_2 > 6.65$ kPa

  E. Hypothermia is an exclusion criteria for BSD

Q 2. **Concerning post-operative surgical site infections:**

  A. Deep infections may occur more than 6 months after implantation of a prosthesis

  B. Clean wounds are associated with infection rates of about 3%

  C. The most common pathogen is *Staphylococcus aureus*

  D. To reduce wound infections the operative site should be shaved the night before surgery

  E. Latex drains reduce the rate of infection following abdominal surgery

Q 3. **Fat embolism:**

  A. Is more common after open than closed fractures

  B. Leads to the fat embolism syndrome (FES) in 20% of cases

  C. Is commonly seen in patients with severe acute pancreatitis

  D. Occurs during the reaming process of intramedullary nailing

  E. Causes hypoxaemia and hypercarbia

Q 4. **Characteristics of the FES are:**

   A. Pulmonary insufficiency
   B. Thrombocytosis
   C. Conjunctival haemorrhages
   D. Petechial rash
   E. Cerebral signs

Q 5. **The following are normal paediatric vital signs:**

   A. Respiratory rate (RR) 40 in a 9 month old girl
   B. Heart rate (HR) 120 in a 4 year old girl
   C. Systolic BP 80 mmHg in a 7 year old boy
   D. HR 60 in a 10 year old girl
   E. Systolic BP 60 mmHg in a 2 year old boy

Q 6. **The following are required in the UK to confirm BSD:**

   A. Two consultants
   B. EEG
   C. Apnoea
   D. Absent gag reflex
   E. A minimum of 24 hours between the two sets of tests

Q 7. **The following are risk factors for nosocomial pneumonia:**

   A. Abdominal surgery
   B. Antibiotic treatment
   C. Intubation
   D. Diabetes
   E. Hypotension

Q 8. **The following organisms are likely to cause lung infections in the intensive care unit (ICU) in the mentioned circumstances:**

   A. *S. aureus* – head injury
   B. *Pseudomonas aeruginosa* – prolonged ventilation
   C. Anaerobes – head injury
   D. *S. aureus* – thoracoabdominal surgery
   E. *Haemophilus influenzae* – tracheotomy

Q 9. **In septic shock, the following antibiotics are appropriate for the suspected site of infection:**

A. GI Tract – clindamycin
B. Surgical wound – vancomycin
C. Lung – piperacillin
D. Urinary tract – penicillin
E. Surgical wound – ceftazidime

Q 1. **The following score highly (2 or more) on the acute physiology and chronic health evaluation (APACHE) scoring system:**

A. Temperature more than 39.2°C
B. Respiratory rate (RR) 24 breaths per minute
C. Heart rate (HR) 105 beats per minute
D. Potassium 5.4 mmol/l
E. Haematocrit 50%

Q 2. **Diamorphine:**

A. Is highly lipid soluble
B. Can be given intrathecally
C. Is excreted primarily by the kidney
D. Has a half life of approximately 30 minutes
E. Is more likely than morphine to produce respiratory depression

Q 3. **Epidural analgesia:**

A. Epidural opioids are five times more potent than intravenous
B. Is associated with decreased respiratory complications
C. May cause cord compression
D. Urinary retention occurs in approximately 10%
E. Hypothesia should be treated with ephedrine and fluids

Q 4. **The following signs would alert a clinician to consider critical care referral:**

A. RR > 30 breaths per minute
B. Mean BP 180 mmHg, HR 100 beats per minute
C. Glasgow coma score (GCS) 7, Pulse 80, BP 130/80 mmHg
D. RR 8 breaths per minute, HR 50 beats per minute
E. Temperature 37.6°C, HR 110 beats per minute

Q 5. **The following factors have been shown to affect outcome in intensive therapy unit (ITU) patients:**

A. Increased age
B. Early diagnosis of the acute condition
C. Severity of the acute illness
D. Physiological reserve
E. Therapy

Q 6. **The following analgesics have the physiological effect stated:**

A. Alfentanil causes sedation
B. Morphine increases bile duct pressure
C. Fentanyl leads to histamine release
D. Fentanyl is an antitussive
E. Morphine increases splanchnic perfusion

Q 7. **Invasive haemodynamic monitoring may be associated with the following complications:**

A. Median nerve neuropathy
B. Very rarely intra-arterial thrombosis
C. Pneumothorax in 10% of central lines
D. Thoracic duct injury demanding surgical intervention
E. Pulmonary artery rupture, during insertion of a pulmonary artery floatation catheter, with a mortality of 50%

Q 8. **Intensive care unit (ICU) scoring systems:**

A. Hospital mortality rate is a useful guide to ICU performance
B. Scoring systems, can be used to decide on optimal treatment for individual patients
C. Risk adjustment is only usually necessary for multi-organ pathology
D. Selection bias may occur due to incomplete validation of data
E. Lead-time bias takes account of any treatment that the patient has had before being admitted to ICU

Q 9. The revised trauma score (RTS):

A. Correlates well with risk of mortality

B. Scores 0–12 by a combination of GCS, mean blood pressure (MBP) and oxygen saturation

C. A score of 12 correlates with over 90% mortality

D. A score of 6 correlates with a 63% survival

E. BP 80/50 mmHg scores 3

Q 10. Scoring systems:

A. APACHE stands for adverse pathology and chronic health evaluation

B. APACHE III is used to guide the most statistically successful treatment

C. SAPS II stands for simplified acute physiology score and has 17 variables

D. APACHE II does not take mechanical ventilation into account

E. APACHE II has more predictive power over individual patient outcome than SAPS II

Q 11. Injury severity scale (ISS):

A. The abbreviated injury score (AIS) is calculated by the sum of the squares of the categories of the ISS

B. AIS lethal dose in 50% (LD 50) is age independent provided patients have the same physiological reserve

C. ISS defines seven anatomical areas

D. In the ISS loss of consciousness for 12 minutes scores 3

E. In the ISS biliary tree injury scores higher than splenic rupture

Q 12. Sedative drugs:

A. Thiopentone is a suitable drug for general sedation in the ICU

B. During propofol infusion, nutritional advice should be sought regarding triphosphopyridine nucleotide (TPN) constitution

C. Etomidate causes muscle twitching

D. Ketamine may be used for rapid sequence induction

E. Midazolam is suitable for long term infusion since it is highly water soluble and does not undergo significant hepatic metabolism

Q 13. Sedative drugs:

A. Propofol and etomidate cause pain on injection
B. Midazolam is the drug of choice for long term sedation since it has a short duration of action
C. Ketamine causes hallucinations
D. Propofol has a duration of action of 2–3 minutes when given by bolus
E. Etomidate does not work in one arm-brain circulation time

Q 14. Analgesic drugs:

A. Morphine and fentanyl have similar elimination half lives
B. Morphine is longer acting than fentanyl
C. Fentanyl is more potent than alfentanil
D. Alfentanil has a longer duration of action than fentanyl
E. Morphine prevents, histamine release by mast cell stabilisation

Q 15. Opioids:

A. May cause chest wall stiffness leading to difficulty with mechanical ventilation
B. Sedation but not pruritus is reversed by naloxone
C. Morphine 3 sulphate is an active metabolite
D. Morphine 6 sulphate is not an active metabolite
E. Cause hypotension by vasodilatation

Q 16. Muscle relaxants:

A. Rocuronium is used for rapid intubation
B. Atracurium is a steroid and should not be used in renal failure
C. Vecuronium may be used in liver failure
D. Vecuronium given as a bolus works within 60 seconds
E. Atracurium is broken down by Hoffmann degradation, which is temperature dependent

Q 17. Suxamethonium:

A. Is structurally related to acetyl choline
B. Causes significant hypokalaemia in burns patients
C. Is metabolised in the liver
D. Causes myalgia
E. Decreases intra-optic pressure (IOP)

Q 18. Physiology of body fluids:

A. Osmolality is the concentration of a solution expressed as osmoles of solute per litre of solution (mosmol/l)
B. Osmolarity is measured by depression of freezing point
C. Toxicity is the osmotic pressure produced by osmotically active particles at selective membranes
D. Semipermeable membranes allow solute but not solvent to pass through
E. Osmolality of plasma is 290 mosmol/l

Q 19. Renal physiology:

A. The kidney is involved in gluconeogenesis
B. Each kidney is made up of twelve thousand nephrons
C. Cortical nephrons have long loops of Henle which pass into the inner medulla
D. Juxtamedullary nephrons account for less than 2% of functional units and are primarily concerned with blood pressure autoregulation
E. The outer medulla has the greatest blood flow reaching 625 ml/min during exercise

Q 20. Renal physiology:

A. Glomerular filtration rate (GFR) is measured by the Fick principle, using the substrate para-amino hippuric acid (PAH)
B. Renal oxygen consumption is large leading to a low renal venous oxygen content
C. The inner medulla is concerned with the countercurrent exchange mechanism and hence has the greatest oxygen consumption

D. The cortex utilises fatty acids in oxidative metabolism

E. The medulla utilises glucose in anaerobic metabolism

Q 21. Renal physiology:

A. Renin is released from the macula densa in the proximal convoluted tubule

B. Renin is a proteolytic enzyme exclusive to the kidney

C. Angiotensin I is an octapeptide

D. Angiotensin II exerts positive feedback on the adrenal cortex

E. Angiotensin II is active in the central nervous system (CNS)

Q 22. Drugs and the kidney:

A. Systemic hypertension causes a diuresis

B. Carbonic anhydrase inhibitors cause a diuresis with low pH and increased ammonia excretion

C. Loop diuretics inhibit Na^+ Cl^- co-transport in the descending loop of Henle causing a large diuresis

D. Thiozide diureticis inhibit Ca^{2+} transport

E. Amiloride is an aldosterone antagonist which reduces K^+ excretion in the distal convoluted tubule

Q 1. Regarding vascular access:

A. Silicone catheters can be thrombogenic

B. Approximately 40% of central venous catheters become colonised with bacteria

C. Vascular catheter related septicaemia occurs in approximately 5% of patients

D. The insertion point for a subclavian catheter is at the junction between the medial 2/3 and the lateral 1/3 of the clavicle

E. The femoral vein lies lateral to the artery in the sheath

Q 2. Regarding intra-cranial pressure (ICP) monitoring:

A. More than 50% of those needing operative treatment of head injuries have rises of ICP more than 20 mmHg

B. ICP > 40 mmHg is associated with neurological abnormalities

C. ICP > 60 mmHg is uniformly fatal

D. Ventricular catheters or subarachnoid bolts are often used

E. ICP monitoring is contra-indicated in infection

Q 3. Complications of tracheotomy:

A. Pneumothorax occurs in upto 5%

B. The inferior jugular vein is most likely to cause bleeding problems

C. Treatment of tracheo-innominate artery erosion (TIAE) requires urgent ligation of the artery

D. Mortality of TIAE, treated rapidly is 10%

E. Approximately 5% of tracheal tubes are accidently dislodges

Q 4. Cricothyroidotomy:

A. The entry point is the cricothyroid membrane, inferior to the cricoid cartilage

B. May be surgical or percutaneous

C. Voice changes occur in half the patients

D. Is associated with subglottic stenosis

E. As an emergency procedure has double the complication rate of an elective procedure

Q 5. The following are complications of arterial line insertion:

A. False aneurysm

B. Haematoma

C. Occlusion

D. Air embolus

E. Thrombosis

Q 6. The following statements concern the internal jugular vein (IJV):

A. Is formed at the jugular bulb and drains blood via the sigmoid sinus

B. Starts its journey through the neck anterior to the carotid artery and ends up lateral to it

C. It runs a straight path from jugular foramen to sternoclavicular joint covered only by carotid sheath and skin

D. Insertion of cannula into the middle third is most comfortable in awake patients

E. Cannulation is less likely to cause arrhythmias than the subclavian vein

Q 7. Vascular access – the following statements concern central line insertion:

A. In patients with head injuries and raised ICP, neutral or head down tilt should be avoided

B. A low approach to the IJV reduces the incidence of side effects

C. The subclavian approach is preferred if there is risk of bleeding to avoid haematoma formation in the neck

D. Placement inadvertently into the external jugular vein (EJV) may not be recognised until the post procedure CXR

E. IJV on the right side is the site of choice since there is less risk of major blood vessel erosion

A 1.   **A.** false   **B.** true   **C.** false   **D.** true   **E.** true

Ventricular tachycardia (VT) suggests either peri-operative myocardial damage or ongoing myocardial ischaemia.

Low urine output requires fluid loading, then dopamine (2 µg/kg/min) before a loop diuretic.

Surgery 1996 14: 4; 78–81   **SCC** pp 49–55

A 2.   **A.** false   **B.** false   **C.** false   **D.** true   **E.** false

The optimal perfusion pressure is 50–70 mmHg. For open heart surgery the superior vena cava (SVC) and inferior vena cava (IVC) are used for the venous cannula. For closed procedures it is the right atrium. The arterial cannula is usually located in the ascending or proximal arch of the aorta. Cooling is between 12–18°C for circulatory arrest.

Surgery 1996 14: 2; 46–48   **SCC** pp 35–37

A 3.   **A.** true   **B.** true   **C.** false   **D.** false   **E.** true

Blood loss should be <100 ml. New Q waves are indicative of a localised myocardial infarction (MI) and occur in <5%.

      SCC pp 49–55

A 4.   **A.** true   **B.** true   **C.** true   **D.** false   **E.** false

Hypercapnia and acidosis rather than those stated.

Surgery 1996 14: 1; 1–5   **SCC** pp 49–55

A 5.   **A.** false   **B.** true   **C.** true   **D.** false   **E.** false

Hypothermia, metabolic acidosis and peripheral cyanosis are features along with cool, clammy skin, poor capillary refill and a low volume pulse. In extreme circumstances, oliguria is in fact anuria.

SCC pp 15–20

A 6. **A.** true **B.** false **C.** true **D.** true **E.** true

Heparin has low lipid solubility and is metabolised in the liver. The use of heparin in disseminated intravascular coagulation (DIC) is controversial but does happen.

SCC pp 41–46

A 7. **A.** true **B.** true **C.** true **D.** false **E.** false

Placement of a pulmonary artery catheter can be confirmed by the waveform along with pulmonary artery wedge pressure being less than mean pulmonary artery pressure, fluid flushing easily when wedged, and wedged PaO_2 < mixed venous PaO_2.

Wedging is contra-indicated in cases of pulmonary infarction. The femoral vein is not uncommonly used for insertion of a pulmonary artery floatation catheter.

SCC pp 18–20, p 214

A 8. **A.** true **B.** true **C.** true **D.** true **E.** true

Noradrenaline reduces renal blood flow by vasoconstriction.

SCC pp 7–8

A 9. **A.** true **B.** true **C.** false **D.** false **E.** true

Dopamine can increase or decrease cyclic AMP. Alpha effects predominate at higher doses and it is less arrhythmogenic than epinephrine.

SCC pp 6–8

A 10. **A.** false **B.** true **C.** true **D.** false **E.** false

Pulmonary artery occlusion pressure is usually decreased in septic and hypovolaemic shock and increased in cardiogenic shock. Cardiac output falls with hypovolaemic and cardiogenic shock and rises in septic shock, as does blood pressure.

A urine output of 15 ml/hr is indicative of class 3 shock (blood loss 1.5–2 litres)

SCC p 20, pp 29–32

A **11.** **A.** true **B.** false **C.** true **D.** false **E.** false

More than 100 ml of gas needs to be injected to cause significant problems. Fat embolus is much more likely than pulmonary embolus 24 hours after a long bone fracture. Aortic thromboemboli have an impact in the renal arteries or those of the lower limb.

Surgery 2002 20: 1; iii–vii SCC pp 44–46

A **12.** **A.** false **B.** true **C.** false **D.** true **E.** false

Haemodynamic instability is an indication for immediate exploration. Disruption is the most common vascular injury followed by intimal injury. Shunting can be a very useful technique for damage control. Packing is useful for venous rather than arterial injuries.

A **13.** **A.** true **B.** true **C.** false **D.** true **E.** false

Management of WBC mediated reactions is to slow the transfusion and administer antipyretics and antihistamines. Massive transfusion is defined as the transfusion of the entire blood volume in 24 hours.

Surgery 2000 18: 2; 48–53 SCC pp 38–41

A **14.** **A.** false **B.** true **C.** false **D.** false **E.** false

The classification of haemorrhagic shock is essential. Detailed tables can be found on page 30 in *Surgical Critical Care* (GMM Ltd, 2001) or *Surgery* 2000 18: 3; 65–68. Systolic BP is normal in class II, pulse pressure normal or elevated in class I, and confusion present in classes III and IV. Class III shock is 30–40% blood loss and is associated with a urine output of 5–15 ml/hr.

SCC pp 29–32

A **15.** **A.** false   **B.** true   **C.** true   **D.** true   **E.** true

The causes of arrhythmias are:

Physiological:

- Acidosis
- Increased CO_2
- Decreased O_2
- Electrolyte imbalance

Pathological:

- Pain
- Phaeochromocytoma
- MI
- Pulmonary embolus

Pharmacological:

- General and local (toxic dose) anaesthetics
- Inotropes

SCC p 51

A **16.** **A.** true   **B.** true   **C.** false   **D.** true   **E.** true

Supportive electrocardiogram (ECG) changes include right ventricular strain (the S1Q3T3 pattern), right axis deviation, right bundle branch block and atrial fibrillation (AF).

SCC p 22

A **17.** **A.** true   **B.** false   **C.** true   **D.** false   **E.** true

Profuse bleeding.

Coagulation Tests: Increased PT, Increased activated partial thromboplastin time (APTT), Increased thrombin time (TT), Increased fibrin degradation products (FDP), Decreased fibrinogen.

Haematology: Decreased platelets, leucocytosis (with left shift).

SCC pp 47–49

A **18.** **A.** true **B.** false **C.** false **D.** true **E.** false

Hartmann's solution is isotonic and contains 5 mmol/l potassium.

N Saline pH = 5.0.

10% of infused 5% dextrose remains intravascular.

SCC p 140

A **19.** **A.** false **B.** true **C.** false **D.** true **E.** true

VT suggests either peri-operative myocardial damage or ongoing myocardial ischaemia. Low urine output should be managed sequentially by fluid load, dopamine 2 μG/kg/min and then loop diuretic.

Surgery 1996 14: 4; 78–81   SCC pp 49–55

A **20.** **A.** true **B.** true **C.** false **D.** false **E.** true

A blood loss of 250 ml would make the surgeon consider re-exploration, the loss should be <100 ml. New Q waves are indicative of localised MI and occur in less than 5% of patients.

SCC pp 49–55

A **21.** **A.** true **B.** true **C.** true **D.** false **E.** false

Causes of cardiac output can be divided into reduced preload (hypovolaemia, cardiac tamponade, tension pneumothorax, right ventricular dysfunction and positive pressure ventilation); reduced contractility (myocardial ischaemia and damage, arrythmias, hypoxia, hypercapnia and acidosis) and increased after load (vasoconstriction and fluid overload)

Surgery 1996 14: 1; 1–5   SCC pp 51–52

A **22.** **A.** true **B.** true **C.** true **D.** true **E.** true

The following may be measured with a pulmonary artery flotation catheter (PAFC)

■ Right and left side cardiac filling pressures
■ Systemic and pulmonary vascular resistance
■ Mixed venous oxygen saturation

- Pulmonary artery pressure
- Cardiac output
- Core blood temperature
- Drug delivery is also possible

Surgery 2002 20: 3; 54–57   SCC pp 18–20

A 23. A. false   **B.** true   **C.** false   **D.** true   **E.** true

Causes of pulseless electrical activity (PEA) can be:

Primary

- MI
- Drugs (β-blocker, calcium antagonists)
- Electrolyte imbalance (hyperkalaemia, hypocalcaemia)

Secondary

- Tension pneumothorax
- Hypovolaemia
- Cardiac tamponade
- Pulmonary embolus
- Cardiac rupture

SCC p 11, pp 13–14

A 24. A. true   **B.** true   **C.** true   **D.** true   **E.** true

Dopamine stimulates cardiac β-1 receptors especially at doses of 5–10 µg/kg/min. The profound tissue damage of extravasation is mediated by α-1 induced vasoconstriction.

SCC pp 6–7

A 25. A. true   **B.** false   **C.** true   **D.** false   **E.** true

Shock should be treated as volume depletion initially. PAFC are often necessary. Vasoactive agents maintain mean arterial pressure. Norepinephrine improves renal function.

SCC pp 29–32

A 26. A. true   **B.** true   **C.** false   **D.** false   **E.** true

Cardiac output (CO) = stroke volume (SV) × heart rate (HR)

It can be corrected for body surface area, when it is called the cardiac index (normal range 2.5–4 l/min/m^2). An increase in filling pressure or preload causes an increase in ventricular end-diastolic volume. This stretches myofibrils and increases myocardial contractility and hence cardiac output. This relationship between myofibril pre-stretching and myocardial contractility is called Starling's Law.

SCC pp 3–11

A 27. A. true   **B.** false   **C.** true   **D.** true   **E.** true

About 80% of total blood volume is contained within the 'low pressure' systemic veins, right heart and pulmonary circulation. Only about 20%, therefore, is in the systemic arterial circulation.

A low central venous pressure (CVP) indicates hypovolaemia. A raised CVP may be caused by volume overload (heart, renal or hepatic failure), pulmonary hypertension, cardiac tamponade, constrictive pericarditis, tricuspid valve disease, or SVC obstruction.

The central control of the circulation is effected by the medullopontine region of the brain. It receives nervous impulses from stretch or pressure receptors in the aorta and carotid sinus, and in the vena cava, atria and left ventricle. An acute increase in blood pressure increases the rate of afferent impulses and causes an increase in vagal discharge resulting in reduced myocardial contractility, and a reduction in sympathetic discharge causing vasodilatation and reduced peripheral resistance. Conversely, an acute fall in blood pressure results in opposite homeostatic responses.

SCC pp 3–11

A 28. A. true   **B.** true   **C.** true   **D.** true   **E.** true

The preload or filling pressure of the right heart is right atrial pressure. That of the left heart is left atrial pressure. Assuming there is no valve disease, atrial pressure equates to ventricular end-diastolic pressure. There is a direct relationship between filling pressure or preload and myocardial contractility. An increase in preload results in an increase in ventricular end-diastolic volume and an increase in the amount of myofibril stretch at the onset of systole. This results in an increase in myocardial contractility.

This relationship can be used to optimise cardiac output in low output states when the administration of fluid with pulmonary artery occlusion pressure (PAOP) monitoring may increase cardiac output. It should be noted, however, that the response is reduced when ventricular function is impaired and that the over-administration of fluid may increase pulmonary venous pressure enough to precipitate pulmonary oedema.

SCC pp 3–11

A 29. A. true **B.** false **C.** true **D.** true **E.** true

Afterload is determined by the aortic valve, peripheral vascular resistance and compliance of the major vessels. There is a direct relationship between afterload and peripheral vascular resistance. At any given preload, decreasing the afterload increases stroke volume.

Cardiac work/beat = stroke work = stroke volume × mean aortic pressure.

A reduction in afterload generally decreases myocardial oxygen demand.

SCC pp 3–11

A 30. A. true **B.** true **C.** true **D.** true **E.** true

The blood oxygen content or amount of oxygen bound by haemoglobin is determined by the haemoglobin concentration and saturation. Cardiac output, haematocrit and local vasomotor tone determine tissue blood flow. Pyrexia, decreasing pH, and increasing concentrations of 2,3-diphosphoglycerate (2,3-DPG) generated by glycolysis shift the oxyhaemoglobin dissociation curve to the right, reducing haemoglobin affinity for oxygen and favour oxygen release to the tissues.

SCC pp 76–78

A 31. A. false **B.** true **C.** false **D.** false **E.** true

Epinephrine and dobutamine are positive inotropes acting at cardiac β-receptors. Myocardial contractility is reduced by hypoxia, acidosis and sepsis. Nitrates are neutral but may improve myocardial contractility indirectly in patients with coronary artery disease through coronary vasodilatation and increased myocardial perfusion. Nitrates also cause peripheral vasodilatation, causing a reduction in preload and pulmonary venous pressure, which is beneficial in heart failure.

SCC pp 3–4, pp 6–8

A 32. A. false **B.** true **C.** false **D.** false **E.** false

Activation of the sympathetic nervous system increases heart rate which (in the early stages of heart failure) compensates for the reduced stroke volume (CO = SV × HR). Reduced renal perfusion results in activation of the renin-angiotensin-aldosterone (RAA) system, which causes sodium and water retention and contributes to the increase in venous pressure seen in heart failure.

The increase in venous pressure (preload) and associated ventricular end-diastolic volume increases myofibril stretching and results in an increase in myocardial contractility (Starling's Law). Activation of the sympathetic nervous system and the RAA system both cause vasoconstriction.

SCC pp 4–5

A 33. A. true **B.** true **C.** true **D.** false **E.** false

As stroke volume decreases, ventricular end-diastolic volume and hence muscle fibre pre-stretching is increased. Through Starling's Law, myocardial contractility is increased. The increase in left ventricular diastolic pressure causes an increase in left atrial pressure reflected in an increase in pulmonary artery occlusion pressure (PAOP). Increased sympathetic activation causes vasoconstriction and an increase in systemic vascular resistance (SVR).

SCC pp 3–5

A 34. A. false **B.** true **C.** false **D.** false **E.** true

The CVP, reflected clinically by the jugular venous pressure (JVP), is most commonly raised due to volume overload (heart failure, renal failure, hepatic failure). Other causes include pulmonary hypertension (e.g. pulmonary embolism (PE), hypoxic lung disease), tricuspid regurgitation, and SVC obstruction when the JVP has a fixed wave form. In cardiac tamponade and constrictive pericarditis, Kussmaul's sign may be present, when the JVP rises on inspiration compared with the normal fall on inspiration. Sepsis is characterised by a vasodilated state so there is usually relative hypovolaemia.

SCC pp 16–18

A 35. **A.** false **B.** true **C.** true **D.** true **E.** true

The subclavian vein traverses anterior to the apex of the lung. Risk of pneumothorax is therefore greater with this approach compared with the internal jugular approach. Nevertheless, a pneumothorax should be excluded by a chest X-ray after either approach.

The risk of accidental arterial puncture exists with both subclavian and internal jugular approaches. The subclavian artery, however, cannot be compressed effectively after accidental puncture. In patients with clotting abnormalities or thrombocytopenia, these should be corrected prior to central line insertion. If vascular access rather than CVP monitoring is required in these patients, cannulation of the femoral vein is safer as haemostasis after accidental puncture of the femoral artery is usually rapidly obtained. CVP monitoring measures right heart preload/filling pressure. This may not reflect the filling pressure of the left heart when there is disparity between left and right heart function e.g. left heart failure, pulmonary hypertension (PE, hypoxic lung disease).

SCC pp 16–18

A 36. **A.** true **B.** false **C.** false **D.** true **E.** true

PAOP is measured by temporary occlusion of a pulmonary artery branch by a balloon flotation catheter. It does not require radiological screening as the balloon-tipped catheter is flow-directed through the right heart to the pulmonary artery and so can be performed in the high dependency unit (HDU) setting. The position of the catheter is identified from the pressure waveform transduced from the catheter tip. Occlusion of a pulmonary artery by the inflated balloon means that only the low-pressure pulmonary veins lie between the catheter tip and the left atrium.

The balloon should be inflated prior to the advancement of the catheter into the pulmonary artery when measuring the PAOP.

Inflation of the balloon within a pulmonary artery branch can cause rupture of the vessel with haemoptysis and occasionally death. The balloon should be deflated after measurement of PAOP otherwise pulmonary infarction can result. Other complications include knotting of the catheter, sepsis, and balloon rupture. Arrhythmias are common but almost invariably transient during advancement of the catheter through the right heart.

SCC pp 17–19

A 37. **A.** false **B.** false **C.** true **D.** false **E.** false

PAOP is a reflection of left atrial pressure, the filling pressure of the left heart. It is the most useful objective measure of volume status in patients in whom this remains uncertain after clinical assessment and CVP measurement.

Adult respiratory distress syndrome (ARDS) is characterised by pulmonary oedema in the presence of a low or normal PAOP. Septic shock is characterised by vasodilatation and PAOP is usually low.

SCC pp 17–19

A 38. **A.** false **B.** true **C.** true **D.** true **E.** false

The two most useful methods of quantifying cardiac output in the HDU setting are by thermodilution and oesophageal Doppler. In thermodilution, 10 ml cold crystalloid is injected into the right atrial port of a pulmonary artery catheter. A thermistor at the catheter tip measures the resultant transient temperature decrease in the pulmonary artery. The area under the fall in temperature against time curve correlates with cardiac output, which is calculated by computer.

The oesophageal Doppler probe measures the velocity of blood flow within the descending thoracic aorta. The area within the velocity-time waveform multiplied by the aortic cross-sectional area (obtained from a nomogram based upon age, height and weight) is aortic blood flow, from which cardiac output can be derived.

Using the Fick principle,

$$CO = \frac{\text{oxygen consumption}}{\text{arteriovenous oxygen content difference}}$$

The main difficulty is an accurate measurement of oxygen consumption, so oxygen consumption is often assumed on the basis of age, gender and body surface area (Indirect Fick method). The additional variables required to calculate arterial and mixed venous oxygen content are haemoglobin concentration, and oxygen saturation in arterial blood and mixed venous (pulmonary artery) blood.

SCC pp 18–20

A **39.** **A.** true **B.** false **C.** true **D.** false **E.** true

Normal PAOP: 4–12 mmHg. Raised values indicate volume overload or mitral valve disease.

Normal SVR: 700–1600 dyn s/cm^5. Low values indicate a vasodilated state such as in septic shock or the systemic inflammatory response syndrome. Raised values occur in hypovolaemia, heart failure and cardiogenic shock.

SCC pp 18–20

A **40.** **A.** true **B.** true **C.** false **D.** false **E.** true

Cardiogenic shock is characterised by a low cardiac output, and raised PAOP and SVR. The raised PAOP reflects the elevated left ventricular end-diastolic and left atrial pressures that accompany left ventricular dysfunction. The raised SVR reflects sympathetic activation, which causes vasoconstriction. The most common cause of cardiogenic shock is acute MI. Other causes include arrhythmias, myocarditis, valve disease including endocarditis, aortic dissection and myocardial depression due to drugs, sepsis and hypoxia.

Management involves monitoring of cardiac rhythm, and invasive blood pressure and CVP monitoring. Measurement of PAOP may be indicated if volume status remains uncertain. Oxygen, intravenous diuretics, and inotropes are invariably required. Intra-aortic balloon pumping (IABP) may be indicated, particularly when there is a potentially correctable cause such as acute mitral regurgitation due to papillary muscle rupture, or ventricular septal defect (VSD) complicating MI.

SCC pp 29–32

41. A. true **B.** false **C.** false **D.** false **E.** false

Septic shock is most commonly caused by gram-negative sepsis (*E. coli*, Meningoccocus) or *Staphylococcus aureus*. Endotoxins cause vasodilatation and increased capillary permeability resulting in hypotension and leakage of fluid from the capillary bed. Cardiac output is usually increased but may be low once metabolic acidosis has supervened. Vasodilatation results in a low SVR. Management includes treatment of the underlying cause (e.g. surgery for intra-abdominal sepsis, antibiotics), correction of hypovolaemia and vasoconstrictive inotropes such as noradrenaline.

SCC pp 29–32

42. A. false **B.** false **C.** true **D.** true **E.** true

The P wave represents atrial depolarisation that triggers atrial contraction and therefore occurs in diastole. There is an inherent delay in conduction as it passes through the atrioventricular node, reflected by the PR interval, which allows the ventricle to fill prior to ventricular contraction. Ventricular depolarisation is reflected by the QRS complex and ventricular repolarisation by the T wave.

Prolongation of the PR interval >200 ms is called 1st degree heart block and reflects delayed conduction through the atrioventricular node. It may reflect a high vagal tone in young, fit adults, or can be caused by MI, β-blockers, calcium channel blockers, hypothyroidism, hypothermia, or age-related degeneration of the conducting system. In isolation, it requires no treatment.

SCC pp 20–22

43. A. true **B.** true **C.** true **D.** false **E.** true

It should be remembered that myocardial ischaemia is not the only cause of ST depression. Left ventricular hypertrophy can cause ST depression and T wave inversion in the inferolateral leads, when it is commonly referred to as a 'strain pattern'. Digoxin may give rise to 'reversed tick' ST depression in the absence of toxicity. Left bundle branch block results in abnormal ventricular depolarisation (broad QRS complex) and repolarisation (giving rise to ST depression and T wave inversion in the lateral leads).

SCC pp 20–23

A 44. **A.** true **B.** true **C.** true **D.** true **E.** true

The characteristic ECG change of MI is ST elevation, though this may also be caused by pericarditis and left ventricular aneurysm. The ECG may, however, be normal or reveal only minor ST/T wave changes. Left bundle branch block may be caused by anterior MI. Complete heart block is relatively common in inferior MI, when it can usually be managed expectantly. Insertion of a temporary pacing wire is indicated when complete heart block occurs in association with anterior MI.

SCC pp 22–23

A 45. **A.** false **B.** true **C.** false **D.** true **E.** false

The diagnosis of post-operative MI may be difficult, particularly after cardiac surgery because creatine kinase is released from traumatised skeletal muscle, and handling of the heart may cause minor ECG changes. Creatinine kinase MB is more specific, but troponin T or I are the most specific markers of myocardial injury.

Cardiac monitoring is mandatory in the first 36 hours after MI as potentially fatal but treatable ventricular tachyarrhythmias occur most commonly early after MI. Thrombolytic therapy is contra-indicated within 6 weeks of major surgery, but aspirin improves prognosis to a similar extent and should be administered in suspected MI. Nitrates do not influence prognosis but are useful for the treatment of continuing chest pain or associated left ventricular failure.

SCC pp 49–55

A 46. **A.** false **B.** true **C.** true **D.** false **E.** true

Both a VSD and mitral regurgitation due to papillary muscle rupture cause a new pansystolic murmur after MI, often associated with cardiogenic shock and so may be confused clinically. Left ventricular pressure is higher than right ventricular pressure so blood passes through the VSD from the left to right ventricle and pulmonary blood flow is increased. The diagnosis can normally be made by transthoracic echocardiography. If cardiac catheterisation is performed, a 'step-up' in oxygen saturation is demonstrated in the right ventricle and pulmonary artery compared with the right atrium as the blood passing from left to right ventricle is oxygenated. Management may be conservative for a small VSD without haemodynamic compromise, or involve supportive measures including IABP and inotropes prior to surgical closure.

SCC pp 49–55

A 47. A. true **B.** true **C.** true **D.** true **E.** true

A small PE may result in no abnormal physical signs or changes on the ECG, so clinical suspicion must be high, particularly in those at risk e.g. post-operative patients, the immobile, those with heart failure or malignancy. Obstruction of a major pulmonary artery branch causes an increase in right-sided heart pressures with elevation of the JVP and dilatation of the right ventricle on echo. Hypoxia and hyperventilation producing a low pCO_2 (type I respiratory failure) are typical of a large PE.

SCC pp 45–46

A 48. A. true **B.** false **C.** true **D.** true **E.** false

Risk of PE is increased by pelvic and lower limb surgery through trauma to the iliac and femoral veins, a substrate for deep vein thrombosis. The risk of thromboembolism associated with malignancy is multifactorial and includes venous compression by tumour, release of prothrombotic mediators, dehydration and immobility. Other risk factors for thromboembolism include heart failure, polycythaemia and prothrombotic conditions e.g. factor V Leiden and factor C & S deficiency.

SCC pp 45–46

A 49. A. true **B.** true **C.** false **D.** true **E.** true

Post-operative pulmonary oedema is commonly caused by pre-existing left ventricular dysfunction, peri-operative myocardial ischaemia or infarction, or overly aggressive intravenous fluid administration, but may be non-cardiogenic in origin (ARDS), particularly in the setting of sepsis or after cardiopulmonary bypass (CPB).

In patients who chronically retain CO_2 (most commonly in chronic obstructive pulmonary disease (COPD)), treatment with high-flow oxygen may remove their hypoxic drive to ventilation resulting in hypoventilation and progressive type II respiratory failure. Nevertheless, it is the hypoxia associated with pulmonary oedema that is acutely life-threatening and this must be rapidly corrected. The development of hypercapnia may require non-invasive or invasive ventilatory support. Intravenous opiate acts as a venodilator reducing pulmonary venous pressure, and as an anxiolytic.

SCC pp 4–5, pp 32–36

A 50. **A.** false **B.** false **C.** true **D.** true **E.** false

The patient should be nursed sitting up. High flow oxygen, intravenous opiate, diuretic and nitrate should be administered. Opiates act as venodilators and anxiolytics. Intravenous frusemide is also a venodilator in addition to its diuretic properties. Nitrates are venodilators, reducing preload and pulmonary venous pressure. β-blockers and angiotensin converting enzyme (ACE) inhibitors improve prognosis in chronic heart failure, but their introduction should be delayed until acute pulmonary oedema has been treated.

SCC pp 32–36

A 51. **A.** true **B.** false **C.** true **D.** false **E.** true

Hypovolaemia is probably the commonest cause of hypotension after surgery so volume status must be assessed, including review of fluid balance charts. Hypovolaemia is often multifactorial with 'nil by mouth', fluid losses from vomiting, drains, fistulae and intra-abdominal sequestration contributing. Post-operative patients are at risk of PE, which may cause hypotension through obstruction of blood flow through a major pulmonary artery. Sepsis causes hypotension through vasodilatation. Treatment is through treating the cause e.g. laparotomy for intra-abdominal sepsis, volume replacement, antibiotics, and inotropes.

SCC pp 49–55

A. true   **B.** true   **C.** true   **D.** true   **E.** true

The cause of hypotension after cardiac surgery may be obvious, e.g. from haemorrhage apparent from drain blood loss, which requires surgical exploration. Cardiac tamponade should be suspected when hypotension occurs in the presence of raised venous pressure. Transthoracic echo (TTE) is the initial investigation, but transoesophageal echo (TOE) may be required to identify compressive thrombus localised around the right atrium. Left ventricular dysfunction may be present pre-operatively and is compounded by peri-operative myocardial ischaemia, arrhythmias, hypoxia and acidosis. Heart block and bundle branch block are common, particularly after valvular surgery, due to damage to the conducting system. External pacing wires are placed at surgery and allow expectant management awaiting spontaneous return of normal conduction, but permanent pacemaker insertion is indicated if advanced heart block persists after 7–10 days. CPB is associated with a systemic inflammatory response due to activation of inflammatory mediators as blood passes through the 'foreign' extra-corporeal circuit. This is usually a self-limiting process but can progress to systemic inflammatory response syndrome (SIRS).

SCC pp 49–55

A 53. **A.** true   **B.** true   **C.** false   **D.** false   **E.** false

AF occurs in 20–40% patients after coronary bypass grafting and is still more common after valve replacement. AF is characterised by the absence of P wave activity and the QRS complexes are irregular (except when complete heart block coexists). The arrhythmia is usually self-limiting after cardiac surgery, assuming pre-operative sinus rhythm. Nevertheless, its occurrence prolongs hospital stay and increases use of resources as spontaneous cardioversion, ventricular rate control and/or warfarinisation is achieved.

SCC pp 49–55

A 54. **A.** true   **B.** true   **C.** true   **D.** true   **E.** true

Post-operative AF is often self-limiting. However, its occurrence may cause troublesome palpitation or promote myocardial

Cardiovascular System

Answers

ischaemia or heart failure. Persistent AF is associated with an increased incidence of thromboembolic stroke. The appropriate management strategy is dependent upon whether haemodynamic compromise is present and on the ventricular rate. If significant haemodynamic compromise is thought to be caused by the new occurrence of AF, then DC cardioversion should be performed. The asymptomatic patient can be managed expectantly, with ventricular rate control until the return of sinus rhythm. Digoxin, β-blockers and verapamil can be used for rate control. If the AF persists, cardioversion should be considered. This can be performed without anticoagulation if the onset of AF occurred within 48 hours as the risk of left atrial thrombus formation is low within this time-frame. Thereafter, 4 weeks of warfarin prior to cardioversion (as an outpatient) is recommended. Cardioversion can be achieved electrically or pharmacologically using agents such as amiodarone. All patients with persistent AF, except those aged <65 years with lone AF, should be considered for warfarin to prevent stroke.

SCC pp 4–5, pp 49–51

A 55. A. true **B.** true **C.** true **D.** true **E.** true

Conduction disorders including complete heart block occur due to damage to the conducting system at surgery. The conduction disorder may be permanent or resolve spontaneously. Second or third degree heart block persisting after 7–10 days requires insertion of a permanent pacemaker.

Endocarditis occurring in the early post-operative period is most commonly caused by coagulase-negative Staphylococci and Staphylococcus aureus. CPB is associated with a systemic inflammatory response due to activation of inflammatory mediators as blood passes through the extra-corporeal circuit. It is usually self-limiting but may cause multi-system failure. When cardiac tamponade occurs as an early complication of cardiac surgery, it usually requires surgical drainage. Neurocognitive impairment is of multifactorial aetiology with factors including CPB, aortic cross-clamping, and thromboembolic events contributing.

SCC pp 49–55

A. false   **B.** true   **C.** true   **D.** false   **E.** false

Hypotension and a raised jugular venous or central venous pressure should raise the suspicion of cardiac tamponade. Cardiac tamponade may result in an increase in the venous pressure on inspiration (Kussmaul's sign) rather than the usual decrease. Pulsus paradoxus (a decrease in systolic blood pressure >10 mmHg during normal inspiration) may be present. Both physical signs reflect the increased intra-pericardial pressure that compresses the heart. The increased venous return that usually occurs on inspiration is constrained causing an increase in right-sided pressures. The atrial and ventricular septae are pushed to the left reducing left ventricular stroke volume and blood pressure. The diagnosis is usually made by transthoracic echo. TOE may be required to demonstrate localised effusion or clot that can occur due to pericardial adhesions after surgery. Management of tamponade early after surgery is usually surgical drainage because the presence of adhesions and thrombus make needle aspiration impractical. Corrigan's sign is a sign of aortic regurgitation and pulsus alternans is a sign of severe impairment of left ventricular function.

SCC pp 49–55

A 57. **A.** false   **B.** false   **C.** false   **D.** true   **E.** true

Pericardiocentesis is indicated in the absence of tamponade when the diagnosis of pericardial effusion is uncertain. Pericardial fluid should be sent for protein concentration, microscopy and culture including TB, cytology, and rheumatoid factor. Malignant disease is a common cause of pericardial effusion and pericardiocentesis may be indicated for diagnosis, treatment of symptoms (typically breathlessness) in the absence of frank tamponade, or tamponade. Such effusions frequently reaccumulate, however, when a pericardial window should be considered. Pericardiocentesis is usually performed by the subxiphoid approach with the patient reclining at 45 degrees. The aspiration needle is advanced towards the left scapula. Echo and X-ray screening can both be used to guide needle placement within the pericardial space. Complications include laceration of a coronary artery or vein or cardiac chamber, vasovagal reactions, arrhythmias, and penetration of the stomach, colon or lung.

SCC p 14, pp 227–228

Cardiovascular System

Answers

A **58.** **A.** true **B.** true **C.** true **D.** false **E.** false

Native valve endocarditis at the aortic site and prosthetic valve endocarditis are most commonly associated with abscess formation. Abscess formation should be suspected if pyrexia and raised inflammatory markers persist after appropriate antibiotic therapy. New-onset conduction disorders are not sensitive but are relatively specific (about 85%) markers for abscess formation. Aortic root abscess is an indication for aortic valve replacement and abscess ablation. Abscesses are usually defined by transoesophageal rather than transthoracic echo.

SCC p 27

A **59.** **A.** true **B.** false **C.** true **D.** true **E.** false

The indications for surgery in endocarditis are haemodynamic compromise due to valve dysfunction, failure of appropriate antibiotic therapy to eradicate infection as indicated by persistent fever and raised inflammatory markers, aortic root abscess, an unstable prosthesis, and recurrent emboli from an infected valve. Although prosthetic valve endocarditis is not an absolute indication for redo valve replacement, it is uncommon for infection to be eradicated from a prosthetic valve by antibiotic therapy alone. If infection is successfully eradicated by antibiotic therapy with little resultant valve dysfunction, a conservative approach to management can be pursued.

A **60.** **A.** false **B.** true **C.** true **D.** true **E.** false

Aortic dissection is thought to begin with a tear in the aortic intima, which exposes a diseased media to blood at systemic arterial pressure. The classical histological change seen in Marfan's syndrome is cystic medial necrosis. Other conditions that predispose to aortic dissection are hypertension, bicuspid aortic valve, coarctation, Ehlers-Danlos syndrome, Noonan and Turner syndromes, pregnancy and trauma, either external chest trauma or internal trauma from a cardiac catheter or balloon pump. There are a number of classifications. The most important feature is whether the ascending aorta is involved. The commonly used Stanford classification has a type A dissection involving the ascending aorta, while a type B dissection does not involve the ascending aorta.

Aortic dissection usually presents with pain, classically tearing in character. Other symptoms and signs depend upon the location of the dissection and involvement of major arterial branches. Signs may include reduced or absent pulses, aortic regurgitation, hemi- or paraplegia.

In type A (proximal) dissections, aortic regurgitation may result either from detachment of an aortic leaflet or dilatation of the aortic root. In 1–2% cases, a proximal dissection flap involves the ostium of a coronary artery (more commonly the right) causing MI. Extension of the dissection into the abdominal aorta may compromise one or both renal arteries or the iliac arteries.

Pleural effusions are common, usually left-sided, and may arise either secondary to an inflammatory reaction around the involved aorta or by a transient leak from a descending dissection. Pericardial effusion may also result from an inflammatory reaction or from haemorrhage into the pericardial space from the dissected aortic root.

A **62.** **A.** false **B.** true **C.** true **D.** false **E.** false

The diagnostic investigations for aortic dissection are MRI, contrast-enhanced CT scanning, TOE and aortography. MRI has a near 100% sensitivity and specificity for the detection of aortic dissection, and does not require the use of ionising radiation or contrast. However, availability of scanners remains limited, and monitoring of and access to unstable patients is compromised in the MRI suite. CT scanning is available at most institutions and is completed more rapidly than MRI. Sensitivity and specificity are about 90%, with higher values for spiral CT scanning. TTE has a low diagnostic sensitivity and specificity, but is readily available, performed at the bedside and provides important information about aortic root size, presence of aortic regurgitation and pericardial effusion, and left ventricular function. TOE has a sensitivity and specificity of about 95% for the diagnosis of aortic dissection. In unstable patients, it should be performed in the anaesthetised patient in the operating room. The introduction of non-invasive diagnostic modalities has seen aortography used less frequently. The procedure is invasive, requires the use of potentially nephrotoxic contrast, carries risks of thromboembolic events, vascular complications, and of entering the false lumen with catheters.

A 63. **A.** false **B.** true **C.** true **D.** true **E.** true

TTE is readily available, non-invasive and provides real-time imaging making it ideal for the assessment of the critically-ill patient. Image quality, however, is often limited in obese patients, those with COPD, and in ventilated patients. TOE can be performed safely in the intubated patient and generally provides superior image resolution. Indications include the diagnosis of aortic dissection or aortic injury, source of embolus, and atrial septal defect. Intra-operative indications include the assessment of mitral valve repair and left ventricular function. TOE has greater sensitivity for the diagnosis of endocarditis than TTE, particularly in prosthetic valve endocarditis, and provides additional information regarding complications such as aortic root abscess and fistula formation.

SCC pp 22–28

A 64. **A.** true **B.** true **C.** true **D.** true **E.** true

Dobutamine is a synthetic inotrope that stimulates β-1, β-2 and α-1 receptors. Its positive inotropic action is through stimulation of cardiac β-1 receptors. Stimulation of β-2 receptors in peripheral vessels causes vasodilatation reducing peripheral vascular resistance, at least at low doses, and this contributes to the increase in cardiac output. These favourable effects on peripheral vascular resistance make dobutamine the favoured inotrope in cardiogenic shock, particularly in the setting of ischaemic heart disease. By contrast, dopamine tends to increase peripheral vascular resistance and causes a greater increase in myocardial oxygen demand and heart rate for a given inotropic effect.

SCC pp 6–8

A 65. **A.** true **B.** false **C.** false **D.** true **E.** true

Epinephrine is an endogenous catecholamine that stimulates α- and β-adrenoceptors. It tends to produce vasoconstriction and an increase in afterload, particularly at higher doses. Myocardial oxygen demand therefore tends to be greater than with dobutamine for a given increase in cardiac output, and myocardial ischaemia may be precipitated, particularly in patients with known coronary artery disease. Current advanced life support (ALS) guidelines recommend the administration of epinephrine 1 mg every 3 minutes of cardiopulmonary resuscitation. At this dose, it produces vasoconstriction and increases peripheral vascular resistance, resulting in a relative increase in cerebral and coronary perfusion. If vascular access is not available, epinephrine can be given down the endotracheal tube, when the dose should be doubled.

SCC pp 7–8

A 66. **A.** false **B.** true **C.** true **D.** true **E.** false

Norepinephrine (noradrenaline) has some β-agonist properties, but acts predominantly at α-adrenoceptors and is therefore a potent vasoconstrictor. It is indicated for hypotension associated with low peripheral vascular resistance that persists after correction of hypovolaemia, e.g. septic shock. Dopamine has a dose-dependent action. At low dose (<2 μg/kg/min), it causes vasodilatation of renal and splanchnic arteries through stimulation of dopamine receptors, which may increase urine volume. Despite this, dopamine has not been shown to improve renal function or to improve outcome in renal failure.
At intermediate doses (2–10 μg/kg/min), cardiac output is increased through β-adrenoceptor activation. At higher doses, α-adrenoceptors are activated producing vasoconstriction. Tachycardia tends to be more pronounced than with dobutamine.

SCC pp 7–8

A 67. **A.** false **B.** false **C.** true **D.** false **E.** true

The IABP is positioned via a femoral artery in the descending thoracic aorta with the balloon tip distal to the left subclavian artery. The IABP can be inserted on the ward when the position is checked by chest X-ray, or under radiological screening. The balloon is timed to inflate during diastole and deflate just prior to the onset of systole. Diastolic pressure is augmented and afterload is reduced resulting in increased coronary and cerebral perfusion and a reduction in myocardial oxygen demand. The balloon can be inflated every cardiac cycle or 1:2 or 1:3 cardiac cycles, which allows weaning from the balloon when the patient has stabilised. The 'foreign' balloon within the circulation is a stimulus to thrombus formation so full heparinisation is required.

SCC p 8

A 68. **A.** true   **B.** false   **C.** false   **D.** true   **E.** false

The IABP results in a reduction in afterload and myocardial oxygen demand, and an increase in coronary and cerebral perfusion. In the clinical setting, it is most commonly used as a stabilising measure prior to definitive surgical intervention. Indications for IABP include refractory angina (typically in patients with left main stem disease, severe three vessel disease, or critical vein graft disease prior to coronary bypass surgery), and cardiogenic shock caused by mitral regurgitation or VSD post-myocardial infarction. IABP is contra-indicated in patients with significant aortic regurgitation (which it exacerbates), aortic dissection, aortic aneurysm, and severe peripheral vascular disease. IABP may be complicated by lower limb ischaemia, thromboembolism, balloon rupture or entrapment, sepsis, and haemorrhage related to the anticoagulation that is required. Lower limb ischaemia warrants balloon removal.

SCC p 8

A 69. **A.** true   **B.** true   **C.** false   **D.** true   **E.** true

The first consideration in suspected cardiac arrest is always safety of rescuer and victim from dangers such as traffic, electricity, gas, water, etc. Next check the victim's responsiveness. If he responds, leave him in the position he was found and get help. If he is unresponsive, call for help, turn him onto his back, and open the airway by 'head tilt/chin lift'. Breathing is assessed for no more than 10 seconds. If he is breathing normally, the victim is placed in the recovery position. If he is not breathing, give two slow, effective rescue breaths. Next check for signs of a circulation (normal breathing, movement, presence of a pulse) for no more than 10 seconds. If a circulation is present, continue rescue breathing. If there are no signs of a circulation, initiate chest

compressions at a rate of 100 per minute, with two rescue
breaths for every 15 compressions.

SCC pp 11–15

A 70. **A.** true **B.** false **C.** false **D.** false **E.** true

Basic life support (BLS) implies that no equipment is used during
the resuscitation. Rescue breaths should take about 2 seconds
and should be sufficient to make the chest rise clearly. The chest
should be allowed to fall before giving another rescue breath.
Chest compressions should be performed at a rate of
100 per minute in a ratio of 15 compressions to 2 rescue breaths.
Compressions are performed on the lower half of the sternum
and should depress the sternum 4–5 cm. In BLS, compressions
cease during the rescue breaths. By contrast, in the intubated
patient (ALS) compressions continue uninterrupted for
ventilations. Optimally performed chest compressions achieve
<30% of the normal cardiac output. Forward blood flow is
achieved by direct compression of the heart, and by changes in
intrathoracic pressure with the heart valves preventing backward
flow (the more important mechanism).

SCC pp 11–15

A 71. **A.** false **B.** true **C.** true **D.** false **E.** false

Irreversible brain damage occurs within 3 minutes of circulatory
arrest. BLS aims to slow the rate of deterioration of the brain
and heart until defibrillation (if appropriate) and ALS is initiated.
BLS itself will rarely, if ever, restore an effective cardiac rhythm.
A praecordial thump is indicated only in a witnessed cardiac
arrest when a defibrillator is not immediately to hand, when it
may revert ventricular tachycardia/ventricular fibrillation (VT/VF)
back to a perfusing rhythm. In adults, the most common cardiac
arrest rhythm is VF. The chances of successful defibrillation
decrease by 7–10% per minute. Thus, the cardiac rhythm should
be established at the earliest opportunity and a shock delivered
if pulseless VT/VF is present. Defibrillation should not be delayed
to perform cardiopulmonary resuscitation unless a defibrillator is
not immediately available. Three shocks are given in succession if
there has been no change in rhythm, with energy levels of 200 J,
200 J and 360 J. If pulseless VT/VF persists, then CPR should be
performed for 1 minute prior to reassessment of the rhythm and

pulse. If pulseless VT/VF persists, three further shocks at 360 J each are administered.

Amiodarone is now the antiarrhythmic drug of choice for shock-resistant pulseless VT/VF. It can be administered in a dose of 300 mg after the third unsuccessful shock.

SCC pp 11–15

A 72. A. true **B.** true **C.** false **D.** true **E.** true

During cardiopulmonary resuscitation, the circulation time from the central veins through the heart to the femoral arteries is approximately 30 seconds compared with up to 5 minutes when a peripheral vein is used. Drug delivery during cardiac arrest is therefore optimally achieved via a central vein. Obtaining central venous access in the setting of a cardiac arrest, however, requires considerable skill and peripheral access may have to be accepted.

Epinephrine (adrenaline) 1 mg should be administered every 3 minutes during cardiopulmonary resuscitation. It causes vasoconstriction and increases cerebral and coronary perfusion.

Open chest cardiac massage (resuscitative thoracotomy) is indicated following recent cardiothoracic surgery, in pulseless electrical activity (PEA) following penetrating trauma, in patients with hyperinflated lungs or a fixed rib cage where external chest compression is not possible, and during abdominal or thoracic surgery.

SCC pp 11–15

A 73. A. false **B.** false **C.** true **D.** false **E.** true

When peripheral or central access cannot be gained rapidly, the tracheal route can be used for the administration of certain drugs. These include epinephrine (adrenaline), atropine, lidocaine (lignocaine), naloxone and vasopressin. The dose of the drug should be increased to 2–3 times that of the intravenous dose. Calcium salts, sodium bicarbonate and amiodarone are not suitable for tracheal administration.

SCC pp 11–15

A. true   **B.** true   **C.** true   **D.** false   **E.** true

PEA was formerly known as electromechanical dissociation (EMD). It is characterised by cardiac arrest with an ECG rhythm, other than VT, compatible with a cardiac output (cardiac arrest with VT is pulseless VT and is managed as VF with defibrillation). The ALS algorithm is the same for asystole and PEA, so for the purposes of management they are grouped together as non-VF/VT. Non-VF/VT rhythms carry a worse prognosis than pulseless VT/VF unless a reversible cause can be identified and treated. Cardiopulmonary resuscitation is performed while the recognised causes of PEA are sought. These include the 4 'Hs' and the 4 'Ts': hypoxia, hypovolaemia, hypothermia, and hypo/hyperkalaemia and other metabolic disorders, tension pneumothorax, cardiac tamponade, thromboembolic circulatory obstruction (massive PE), and toxic/therapeutic substances e.g. calcium channel blocker and β-blocker overdose. During cardiopulmonary resuscitation, epinephrine 1 mg should be administered every 3 minutes. In PEA, atropine 3 mg should be administered only if the heart rate on ECG is <60/minute.

SCC pp 11–15

A 1. **A.** true **B.** false **C.** true **D.** true **E.** true

Positive end expiratory pressure (PEEP) increases: Functional residual capacity (FRC), intra-cranial pressure (ICP) compliance, and barotrauma.

SCC p 84, p 94

A 2. **A.** true **B.** false **C.** true **D.** false **E.** true

The features are respiratory rate (RR) > 30 breaths per minute, O_2 saturation < 80%, PaO_2 < 8 KPa, $PaCO_2$ > 7 kPa, dyspnoea, increasing distress, exhaustion, sweating, confusion, vital capacity < 15 ml/kg, FEV_1 (forced expiratory volume) < 10 ml/kg.

SCC pp 79–80

A 3. **A.** true **B.** true **C.** true **D.** true **E.** true

Hyponatraemia can occur with low, normal or high extracellular fluid (ECF) volume. Urine sodium levels help distinguish between the causes.

SCC p 157

A 4. **A.** true **B.** true **C.** true **D.** true **E.** true

All the above plus pneumatoceles, retroperitoneal air and acute lung injury (ALI).

SCC pp 80–86

A 5. **A.** false **B.** true **C.** true **D.** true **E.** true

Hyperthyroidism rather than hypothyroidism can cause respiratory alkalosis. The remainder all can.

SCC pp 74–75

A. false **B.** true **C.** true **D.** true **E.** false

Adult respiratory distress syndrome (ARDS) is characterised by respiratory failure, diffuse alveolar infiltrates on chest X-ray, and a normal or low pulmonary artery occlusion pressure (PAOP). The latter qualification differentiates the condition from cardiogenic pulmonary oedema. ARDS has many possible causes that include septicaemia, cardio-pulmonary bypass, acute pancreatitis, fat embolism, trauma, burns, smoke inhalation, placental abruption and amniotic fluid embolism. ARDS reflects a systemic inflammatory response that is usually associated with multi-organ dysfunction. There is a generalised increase in vascular permeability mediated by inflammatory cytokines. In the lung, this is reflected by alveolar infiltrates comprising fibrin, platelets and inflammatory cells. Subsequent fibroblast activation results in pulmonary fibrosis. Management is supportive while the underlying cause, most commonly sepsis, is treated. Ventilatory support is required. Volume overload should be avoided. There is no evidence that steroids improve prognosis in ARDS. Prostacyclin reduces pulmonary artery pressures, but its role in the management of ARDS remains to be established. Prone ventilation may improve oxygenation.

SCC pp 91–96

A 7. **A.** true **B.** true **C.** true **D.** true **E.** true

Respiratory failure is defined by a $PaO_2 < 8\,kPa$ and is divided into type I when the $PaCO_2$ is normal or low, and type II when the $PaCO_2$ is raised. A number of conditions may cause respiratory failure in the post-operative period. Whether or not respiratory failure occurs depends upon the severity of the condition e.g. pneumonia, and the pre-existing lung function. Those with pre-existing abnormal lung function, most commonly due to chronic obstructive pulmonary disease (COPD), are more likely to develop post-operative respiratory failure since they have less reserve. The commonest post-operative respiratory complication is basal atelectasis. This occurs due to inadequate ventilation and expectoration resulting in retained secretions due to pain, and diaphragmatic splinting due to ileus. It may become complicated by superadded infection. Prevention focuses on adequate analgesia and physiotherapy.

Opiate analgesia may result in (type II) respiratory failure through depression of the respiratory centre. Pulmonary embolism usually causes type I respiratory failure as $PaCO_2$ is low due to hyperventilation to compensate for hypoxia. ARDS may complicate any major surgery, particularly after cardio-pulmonary bypass.

SCC pp 79–80

A 8. **A.** false **B.** false **C.** false **D.** false **E.** true

Central chemoreceptors are located close to the floor of the fourth ventricle, near the respiratory centre in the brainstem. They are sensitive to pH change in the cerebrospinal fluid (CSF) that surrounds them. Hydrogen (H^+) and bicarbonate (HCO_3^-) diffuse slowly between blood and CSF, CO_2 however moves freely CSF is low in protein and buffering capacity is poor. Therefore relatively little increase in CO_2 levels have a profound effect on CSF pH. This pH change is detected by the central chemoreceptors and information relayed to the respiratory centre to increase (for ↑ CO_2) or decrease (for ↓ CO_2) the rate and depth of breathing. CO_2 changes in the CSF is eventually buffered by the slow diffusion of HCO_3^- across the blood brain barrier.

SCC p 60

A 9. **A.** false **B.** false **C.** true **D.** false **E.** true

Peripheral chemoreceptors are sensitive to O_2 and are found in the carotid and aortic bodies. The output from peripheral chemoreceptors increases with hypoxia down to PaO_2 4.4 kPa, below which it remains constant but does not stop. The combined effects of hypercabia and hypoxia are summative central chemoreceptors are located in the ventral medulla. The Hering-Breuer reflex is protective and prevents damage due to volutrauma and barotrauma, by limiting maximal inspiration.

SCC p 60

A 10. **A.** false **B.** true **C.** false **D.** false **E.** false

Total lung capacity is the total volume of air in the lungs at the end of a maximal inspiration. The expiratory reserve volume is usually 1 litre in adults. Closing capacity is the lung volume where small airways begin to collapse on expiration. If this falls below FRC during tidal (normal) ventilation then it will result in hypoxaemia. Total lung capacity is the combination of vital capacity and residual volume, irrespective of atmospheric pressure.

SCC pp 61–62

A **11.** **A.** false   **B.** false   **C.** true   **D.** true   **E.** false

FRC is the volume of air remaining in the lung after tidal expiration, and is usually 2.2 litres in adults. Its importance is as a source of oxygen reserve, which can continue to take place in gaseous exchange between breaths. The relationships between FRC and closing capacity is important since the air mixture in the FRC can only take place in gaseous exchange if the airways are given. Reducing FRC compared with closing capacity therefore leads to hypoxaemia. All manoeuvres that increase lung volume will improve FRC. Regional anaesthesia does not increase FRC *per se* but prevents the further decrease seen with general anaesthesia.

SCC pp 61–62

A **12.** **A.** false   **B.** true   **C.** false   **D.** true   **E.** false

Respiratory compliance is the change in volume (l) per unit change in pressure (kPa). It gives an indication of the amount of work required to expand the lungs during inspiration.
The characteristic sigmoid shaped compliance curve suggests that compliance is decreased at extremes of lung volume i.e., low and high lung volumes. Compliance is reduced at the extremes of age, in the newborn because of the increased tendency for the lung to collapse, and in the elderly because of reduced tissue elasticity. Compliance is reduced by restrictive and obstructive lung disease.

SCC pp 62–64

A **13.** **A.** false   **B.** false   **C.** true   **D.** false   **E.** false

During spontaneous ventilation the majority of the inspired gas is directed to the lower (dependent) parts of the lungs. This is because of the greater negative pressure generated at the base. Compliance is greatest (i.e. steepest part of the curve) in the middle zones (west zones 2 and 3) during spontaneous ventilation. With mechanical ventilation inspired gas is directed preferentially towards the upper (non-dependent) areas of the lungs where compliance is now greatest. More work is required to distend the lower (west zone 4) areas of the lung with positive pressure ventilation, hence they are shown as flat portions of the sigmoid shaped compliance curve. Hypoxic pulmonary vasoconstriction (HPV) is a method whereby blood is directed away from under ventilated areas of the lung, reducing the potential for shunt, and hence hypoxaemia.

SCC p 65

A 14. A. false **B.** false **C.** false **D.** true **E.** false

Shunt refers to areas of the lung which are well perfused but poorly ventilated. Dead space refers to areas of the lung which are well ventilated but poorly perfused. Both lead to arterial hypoxaemia. The arterial hypoxaemia of shunt cannot be corrected by increasing the inspired oxygen concentration alone since the affected areas are poorly ventilated, hence the increased oxygen concentration does not come into contact with blood. Blood supply decreases from the bottom to the top of the lung. Ventilation also decreases but to a lesser degree. This leads to the tendency for the upper parts of the lung to develop increased dead space and lower (dependent) parts of the lung to develop increased shunt. The optimal part of the lung for gaseous exchange is therefore the mid portion (west zones 2 and 3).

SCC p 65

A 15. A. false **B.** false **C.** true **D.** false **E.** false

FEV_1/FVC ratio is usually 0.8. The ratio is usually increased in restrictive conditions since the FVC is often reduced to a larger degree than the FEV_1. The ratio is decreased in obstructive conditions since the FVC remains largely constant but the FEV_1 is often severely reduced. Both restrictive and obstructive conditions may be diagnosed but the results depend on the overall clinical picture and the technique of the patient in obtaining the data. Restrictive conditions can give a normal ratio but the absolute values are usually below the normal range for sex, height and weight. Pulmonary function tests are usually carried out in a laboratory with the use of a spirometer. Peak flow meters are a bedside test to monitor treatment.

SCC pp 65–67

A **16.** **A.** true   **B.** false   **C.** false   **D.** false   **E.** true

The normal range for $PaCO_2$ is 4.4–5.8 kPa. The normal range for PaO_2 (breathing room air) is 10–13 kPa. pH is indirectly proportional to the H^+ content of blood (negative logarithm). Standard bicarbonate (SBC) is a measure of plasma HCO_3^- corrected to a $PaCO_2$ of 5.3 kPa, thus removing the influence of any respiratory effects. Decreasing the temperature of a sample decreases the pH and oxygen content, therefore the H^+ content increases with decreasing temperature. Normal pH at 27°C is 7.25.

SCC pp 67–75

A **17.** **A.** false   **B.** false   **C.** false   **D.** false   **E.** false

Homeostasis involves the maintenance of constant pH, which is essential for cellular function. Acidosis and alkalosis leads directly to cellular dysfunction and end organ damage. The bicarbonate buffer system:

$$H_2O + CO_2 \rightleftharpoons H_2CO_3 \rightleftharpoons H^+ + HCO_3^-$$

accounts for over two thirds of the body's buffering capacity. This is an open buffer system since the components can be varied independently of each other (CO_2 by the lungs and HCO_3^- by the kidneys). Deoxygenated haemoglobin has greater buffering capacity than the oxygenated form. Full compensation of acid-base imbalance will result in return to normal values and does not result in over correction (unless there is another pathological process occurring).

SCC pp 67–75

A **18.** **A.** true   **B.** false   **C.** false   **D.** false   **E.** true

Metabolic acidosis results from increased H^+ levels or decreased HCO_3^- levels. The commonest causes are lactic or keto acidosis, renal failure and diarrhoea. Although blood HCO_3^- levels are low sodium bicarbonate is reserved for severe or unresponsive cases only. Sodium bicarbonate can lead to worsening intracellular acidosis and presents a large sodium and carbon dioxide load, often in situations when the body's excretory mechanisms are over stretched. The main goal of therapy is treatment of the underlying cause and re-hydration. Normal compensation is by hyperventilation. Salicylate poisoning can lead to a mixed picture of metabolic acidosis and respiratory alkalosis.

SCC pp 69–71

A 19. **A.** false **B.** false **C.** false **D.** true **E.** true

This is the clinical picture of diabetic keto acidosis. The metabolic acidosis exists because of the build up of acid in the form of ketones. This is a life threatening condition and the primary concern is to rehydrate the patient with normal saline. As a result of polyuria in the initial stages caused by an osmotic diuresis, the patient may be severely dehydrated and require upto 10 litres of fluid resuscitation. Control of blood sugar is secondary and should be done gradually. Urine output should be monitored carefully.

SCC pp 69–71

A 20. **A.** true **B.** true **C.** true **D.** false **E.** true

This is the clinical picture of metabolic alkalosis. The main causes are loss of H^+ from the kidneys e.g. diuretic therapy, hypokalaemia or mineralocorticoid excess; or H^+ loss from the gut e.g. vomiting. Compensation is by hypoventilation which may result in hypoxia. Normal saline may be indicated for hypochloraemic hypovolaemia associated with vomiting. Urine pH is usually alkaline to prevent further loss of H^+.

SCC pp 71–72

A 21. **A.** false **B.** false **C.** false **D.** true **E.** false

Respiratory acidosis with asthma is a grave sign and may herald respiratory arrest. Airway + Breathing are of primary concern in all patients. In trauma cases the airway should be secured if there is any doubt about the patency or the mechanism for ventilation.

Failure to correct airway or breathing insufficiency early may lead to difficulty later (often when patients, have been moved to less well monitored areas e.g., CT scan). Sodium bicarbonate increases the CO_2 burden and compounds the problem. Pre-existing compensated respiratory acidosis (due to CO_2 retention e.g. in COPD patients) can lead to normal pH with elevated $PaCO_2$. HCO_3^- formed from CO_2 is neutralized by the bicarbonate buffer system, the increased H^+ is excreted in the urine.

SCC pp 72–73

Respiratory System

A 22. A. true   **B.** true   **C.** false   **D.** false   **E.** false

Early pneumonia and ARDS often results in respiratory alkalosis, which may become acidosis as the clinical condition worsens. Respiratory alkalosis is usually driven by hypoxia and therefore oxygen therapy is essential whilst working out the cause. Oxygen therapy may well reverse the respiratory alkalosis by reducing respiratory drive. When occurring in patients with known deep vein thrombosis (DVT) may herald a pulmonary embolus, which can be fatal. The normal compensatory mechanism is to preserve H^+ ions and therefore produce an alkaline urine.

SCC pp 74–75

Answers

A 23. A. true   **B.** false   **C.** false   **D.** true   **E.** false

$$\text{Oxygen delivery } DO_2 = CO \times [(Hb \times {}^{Sat}\!/_{100} \times 1.34) + (PaO_2 \times 0.003)]$$

Although Hb 15 g/dl carries more oxygen than Hb 10 g/dl the reduced viscosity of the latter affords more efficient delivery to the tissues. Oxygen delivery is reduced at altitude because of reduced partial pressure of the inspired air, despite the fact that cardiac output (CO) greatly increases. Because the vast majority of the oxygen carrying capacity is due to its combination with haemoglobin, increasing the inspired oxygen concentration will have little extra effect on oxygen delivery providing that haemoglobin is already fully saturated with O_2. The dissolved fraction is usually negligible and rises relatively little with increased O_2 concentration in the inspired air.

SCC pp 76–78

A 24. **A.** false **B.** false **C.** false **D.** true **E.** true

Carbon monoxide poisoning causes anaemic hypoxia since its high affinity for haemoglobin prevents the usual binding of oxygen molecules. Stagnant hypoxia is due to low CO states and causes high oxygen extraction leading to a lower venous oxygen content. Conversely high venous oxygen content may be seen in conditions with hyperdynamic circulations such as sepsis. Altitude and cyanotic heart disease result in hypoxic hypoxia resulting in reduced haemoglobin saturation and low oxygen partial pressure in blood.

SCC pp 76–77

A 25. **A.** false **B.** false **C.** false **D.** true **E.** false

Post-operative shivering is problematic because the increased muscle movement greatly elevates the body's oxygen requirements. Oxygen therapy is given to satisfy the increased needs of the body and not to stop the shivering. The Hudson mask is a variable performance oxygen delivery system where the oxygen concentration depends on the patient's minute volume and peak inspiratory flow rate (PIFR). At high PIFR room air is entrained leading to a reduction in oxygen concentration delivered to the patient. 10 l/min via the Hudson mask gives an oxygen concentration of 61–73%.

SCC pp 77–78

A 26. **A.** true **B.** false **C.** true **D.** false **E.** true

Venturi masks deliver a constant oxygen concentration independent of the patients respiratory pattern (minute volume and PIFR). The oxygen supply entrains air at a fixed rate via a jet built into the mask. These masks, unlike Hudson masks are colour coded: white (28%), yellow (35%), red (40%) and green (60%). Venturi masks are used when patients require known concentrations of oxygen e.g. COPD patients. Hudson masks are a simpler design and tend to be used for routine post-operative use. Venturi masks are less efficient than Hudson masks since they only entrain a certain amount of room air.

SCC p 78

A **27.** **A.** true   **B.** false   **C.** true   **D.** false   **E.** true

In type I respiratory failure there is hypoxaemia with low or normal $PaCO_2$. In Type II respiratory failure there is hypoxaemia with hypercarbia, leading to respiratory acidosis. Type I failure may be due to early pneumonia or ARDS with hypoxaemia being the precipitant for increased respiratory effort resulting in a respiratory alkalosis. As these diseases progress, so the patient is more likely to develop type II failure as they get exhausted or because of an increased diffusion barrier for gaseous exchange in the lungs. Guillain Barré is a neuromuscular condition believed to be immunologically mediated. This results in a flaccid paralysis of the body, including the respiratory muscles leading to a mechanical failure of ventilation and type II failure.

SCC pp 79–80

A **28.** **A.** false   **B.** false   **C.** false   **D.** false   **E.** true

Whilst both types of respiratory failure are serious conditions requiring urgent medical attention, type I failure is usually driven by hypoxaemia and is associated with less mechanical difficulty in ventilation. Correction of the hypoxia will provide time for diagnosis and clinical prioritisation. Type II failure often requires immediate action to prevent severe ventilatory compromise or even respiratory arrest. In some instances (but not always) type I may be thought of as an earlier stage than type II. Kyphoscoliosis tends to be a mechanical ventilatory failure leading to type II respiratory failure. Although patients with type II failure have tachypnoea their ventilatory excursion is usually inadequate, leading to CO_2 retention. Flail chest leads to mechanical failure of ventilation (type II).

SCC pp 79–80

A **29.** **A.** false   **B.** false   **C.** false   **D.** false   **E.** true

Cyanosis is the blue discolouration of the skin caused by the presence of greater than 5 g/dl of deoxyhaemoglobin. It is possible to have cyanosis without hypoxia in polycythaemic patients and hypoxia without cyanosis in anaemic patients. A lowered level of consciousness is not a reliable sign of respiratory distress *per se*, but in combination with other signs suggests a severe level of hypoxia. Head injuries may lead to tachypnoea and loss of consciousness without respiratory failure. Tachypnoea is also associated with hypovolaemia and the compensation for metabolic acidosis. Tachycardia is associated with a multitude of clinical situations unrelated to respiratory failure. The appearance of intercostal or subcostal recession and tracheal tug are pretty specific signs of respiratory failure with the body using every possible mechanical advantage to improve ventilation.

SCC pp 79–80

A 30. **A.** false **B.** true **C.** false **D.** false **E.** false

The decision to institute respiratory support is often complicated and dependent on several factors. The PaO_2 should be less than 8 kPa on 60% oxygen (not 40%). The $PaCO_2$ level will depend on the patient's pre-morbid level and the use of a general 'cut-off' figure for every patient is not helpful. However for patients without a previous history of respiratory failure or hypercapnoea a $PaCO_2$ above 8 kPa is usually taken as significant. Protection of the lower airway should be instituted in patients with a Glasgow coma score (GCS) less than 8, this will usually also require mechanical ventilation. The presence of a tracheostomy is not an indication for respiratory support in itself.

SCC pp 80–87

A 31. **A.** false **B.** true **C.** false **D.** true **E.** true

Expiration is passive in spontaneous and mechanical ventilation. Pneumothoracies should always be drained prior to intermittent positive pressure ventilation (IPPV), since there is a significant risk of causing tension pneumothorax by increasing the intra-thoracic pressure. HPV is reduced by both IPPV and anaesthesia, increasing the risk of shunt and hypoxaemia. Blood pressure may initially increase due to the increase in intra-thoracic pressure. Acid/base disturbances may result from under or over ventilation.

SCC pp 81–82

A 32. **A.** true **B.** false **C.** true **D.** false **E.** true

IPPV reduces venous return by increasing intra-thoracic pressure. The negative intra-thoracic pressure of spontaneous ventilation acts to 'pump' blood back to the heart. Sedation is usually required since the patient is often intubated, which is stimulating to the gag reflex. Blood pressure may be reduced on correction of acidosis because of lowering endogenous adrenaline levels. Hypercarbia is associated with catecholamine release and hypertension and tachycardia. Glomerular filtration rate is decreased as a result of reduced renal blood flow and CO. The rise in intra-thoracic pressure is transmitted via the venous system to increased intra-cranial pressure. This is often offset however, by the ability to control CO_2 levels and hence intra-cranial volume.

SCC pp 81–82

A 33. A. false   **B.** false   **C.** false   **D.** true   **E.** false

F_IO_2 is the fractional inspired oxygen concentration and should be set to 0.5 (50%) initially. Subsequent adjustment will depend on frequent arterial blood gas sampling. In extreme circumstances the F_IO_2 may be set to 1.0 but this increases the risk of absorption atelectasis and lung collapse. Tidal volume is usually set at 10–12 ml per kg. Oxygen is mixed with air to prevent absorption atelectasis in the intensive care unit (ICU) since nitrous oxide is an anaesthetic. The nitrogen in air being inert is not absorbed in the lungs, thus 'splinting' them open. Asthmatics require longer expiratory times due to the obstructive nature of the condition. PEEP has a number of side effects, mainly on decreasing venous return and is not applied unless required.

SCC pp 81–82

A 34. A. true   **B.** false   **C.** false   **D.** false   **E.** true

The ventilator will deliver a set tidal volume at a set RR. The patient is usually sedated and paralysed with muscle relaxant and makes no respiratory effort. Peak pressure will depend on the patient's respiratory compliance. As compliance reduces so the peak pressure will increase, and enhances the risk of damage to the lungs by barotrauma. This is therefore not a useful mode of ventilation for patients with poor compliance. Since the patient is sedated and paralysed this mode of ventilation is not suitable for weaning.

SCC pp 83–87

A. true   **B.** false   **C.** false   **D.** true   **E.** true

Minute volume is made up of a mixture of mandatory breaths initiated by the ventilator and spontaneous breaths initiated by the patient. This leads to an inconsistency of volume between cycles. Spontaneous and mandatory (machine) breaths are synchronised so that the machine breaths can only be delivered when the patient is not taking a spontaneous breath. This prevents high peak airway pressures and the risk of barotrauma. This is a weaning mode and therefore muscle relaxation is counter-productive, also the patient must be able to initiate a breath. The mixture of spontaneous and mechanical breaths allows a more favourable ventilation to perfusion profile than controlled mandatory ventilation (CMV) which results in much higher intra-thoracic pressures.

SCC pp 83–87

A 36.   **A.** false   **B.** false   **C.** true   **D.** false   **E.** true

Pressure controlled ventilation (PCV) is used when pulmonary compliance is low. The peak pressure and RR are set on the ventilator and the minute volume delivered to the patient will depend on the compliance. Because of the square wave pressure trace the resultant mean airway pressure (MAWP) is higher than the CMV trace for any given peak airway pressure. Since MAWP equates with oxygenation, PCV therefore results in improved oxygen delivery. Muscle paralysis is often required as the patient is fully ventilated and spontaneous activity is not encouraged.

SCC pp 83–87

A 37.   **A.** false   **B.** true   **C.** false   **D.** false   **E.** false

Pressure support ventilation (PSV) is a weaning mode that requires the patients to be completely unparalysed, since they initiate all of the delivered breaths. A level of pressure support is set on the ventilator and the tidal volume delivered to the patient will depend on their lung compliance. The ventilator does not initiate any of the breaths delivered. Sedation is sometimes required because the patient may still be intubated, which stimulates the gag reflex. The level of respiratory support may be reduced as weaning progresses until the patient can breath spontaneously unaided.

SCC pp 83–87

A **38.** **A.** false **B.** true **C.** false **D.** false **E.** true

PEEP is used to prevent collapse of the airway, which leads to hypoxia, during ventilator delivered breaths. Continuous positive airways pressure (CPAP) is used for spontaneous breaths in both intubated (including tracheostomies) and unintubated subjects. Both PEEP and CPAP reduce venous return and consequently reduce CO and blood pressure. Inverse ratio ventilation (IRV) is used to recruit collapsed alveoli in patients on PCV. Expiration is always passive. Since the time allowed for expiration is greatly reduced, respiratory acidosis can occur as the CO_2 rises. This can be an extremely unstable mode of ventilation cardiovascularly since there is little time for venous return during expiration.

SCC pp 80–87

A **39.** **A.** false **B.** true **C.** false **D.** false **E.** false

If the patient continues to need opioids for pain management or to tolerate the endo-tracheal tube (ETT) then they should continue. PCV is not an easy mode to wean from since the patients usually require a large amount of support – but it can be done. Patients should be put onto a T-piece, which offers no protection against airway collapse and no pressure support when the synchronised intermittent mandatory ventilation (SIMV) rate is zero, pressure support $10 \, cmH_2O$ and PEEP $5 \, cmH_2O$. When a patient first goes onto a T-piece it may be desirable to alternate this with periods on the ventilator to maintain alveolar recruitment and prevent collapse.

SCC pp 85–87

A **40.** **A.** false **B.** true **C.** false **D.** false **E.** true

- The correct length for a paediatric ETT is age/2 + 12 cm
- The correct diameter for a paediatric ETT is age/4 + 4 cm
- The correct diameter for an adult female is 7.5–8 mm
- The correct length for adults is 23 cm (male) and 21 cm (female)

Cricoid pressure is also known as Sellicks manouvre and is applied with a force of 40 Newtons vertically downward on the cricoid cartilage. One or two hands may be used and its purpose is to prevent gastric aspiration during induction of anaesthesia as part of a rapid sequence induction technique. This technique is employed in all situations where a full stomach is suspected e.g. emergency surgery or trauma.

SCC pp 90–91

A 41. **A.** false **B.** true **C.** false **D.** true **E.** false

Nasal intubation is mainly practiced in children an ICU. Nasal intubation is better tolerated than oral and does not stimulate the gag reflex to such a large extent. Sedation requirements are therefore much reduced in this group of patients. Nasal intubation requires laryngoscopy just as oral intubation does and is therefore just as cardiovascularly stimulating. Tracheostomy is indicated for prolonged weaning or ventilation and facilitates continued protection of the airway in patients, with impaired pharyngeal reflexes or conscious level. Tracheostomy is not indicated primarily for obesity, although obese patients may fall into the group that have prolonged ventilation and weaning. There may be technical difficulties in securing a tracheostomy in obese patients.

SCC pp 87–91

A 42. **A.** true **B.** false **C.** true **D.** false **E.** true

ARDS is the pulmonary component of the systemic inflammatory response syndrome (SIRS). It is essentially an inflammatory response to a substantial insult. The commonest causes are sepsis and trauma both pulmonary and extra-pulmonary. Other common causes are pancreatitis, haemorrhage and shock, gastric aspiration and associated with massive blood transfusion. Raised intra-cranial pressure leads to neurogenic pulmonary oedema which although giving a similar clinical picture to ARDS has a different pathological process.

SCC pp 91–96

A 43. **A.** false **B.** false **C.** false **D.** false **E.** false

A recent consensus conference has based the definition of ARDS on the presence of the following criteria:

I.   There must be a known precipitating cause
II. The onset of symptoms must be acute
III. There must be new bilateral fluffy infiltrates on the CXR (this may lag behind the clinical picture by 12–24 hours)
IV. There must be no cardiac failure or fluid over load (peak airway pressure (PAWP) must be <18 mmHg)

Although it is likely that the patient will require mechanical ventilation and that they usually have high airway pressures, this does not form part of the defining criteria. In ARDS the $PaO_2 : F_IO_2$ ratio is <40 kPa, but in ALI, a less severe illness the $PaO_2 : F_IO_2$ ratio is >27 kPa, signifying less hypoxaemia.

SCC pp 91–96

A 44. **A.** true **B.** false **C.** true **D.** false **E.** false

The inflammatory response releases mediators such as cytokines, tumour necrosis factor (TNF), platelet activating factor (PAF) and interleukin (IL). These cause capillary endothelial damage leading to increased permeability and a protein rich exudate fills the alveoli. This results in atelectasis and collapse leading to arterial hypoxaemia. Late features are fibroblast proliferation leading to fibrosis and collagen deposition resulting in microvascular obliteration. A fibrosing-alveolitis picture may be seen in some patients but this is a late development.

SCC pp 91–96

A 45. **A.** false **B.** false **C.** false **D.** true **E.** false

Fluids should be given judiciously since the hypoxaemia may be made worse by further alveolar oedema. Concurrent sepsis or hypovolaemia has to be addressed but careful monitoring of central pressures should be observed. A PAFC may be useful for fluid management but is not essential in the treatment of ARDS, the management of which is largely supportive. PAFC's do have an inherent morbidity and mortality attached to their insertion and should be used only when required. The basis of the respiratory support should be to prevent further harm to the good (unaffected) parts of the lung whilst supporting the damaged parts. Therefore moderate hypoxaemia ($PaO_2 > 8\,kPa$) and permissible hypercapnoea ($PaCO_2$ 10–15 kPa) may be tolerated if there is no cerebral oedema, acidosis or cardiovascular compromise. High peak airway pressures are avoided to protect the lung.

SCC pp 91–96

A **46.** **A.** false   **B.** true   **C.** true   **D.** false   **E.** false

PEEP is usually required to move the lower part of the compliance curve to a more favourable (steeper part of the curve) position. PEEP prevents the collapse of recruited alveolar units in the lung, so reducing hypoxaemia. FRC acts as an oxygen store and when increased improves oxygenation. IRV increases MAWP which optimises oxygenation but reduces CO_2 removal because of the reduced expiratory time, therefore overall gas exchange is not optimised. Nitric oxide is also known as endothelial derived relaxant factor and is a potent vasodilator. When given by nebuliser it passes to those 'healthy' unaffected lung units and improves the bloodflow thus reducing dead space and improving hypoxia. If given intravenously however it has a general effect, worsening shunt in areas of the lung that are damaged and therefore perfused but not adequately ventilated.

SCC pp 91–96

A **47.** **A.** false   **B.** false   **C.** true   **D.** true   **E.** false

Prognosis is affected by increasing age, significant past medical history and the nature of the precipitating event. Sepsis has the highest mortality and polytrauma the lowest. Early deaths are usually related to the precipitating cause, whereas late deaths are associated with multi-organ failure. Pneumothorax is common with high PAWP and damaged lung tissue. Once drained ventilation may be difficult because the air leak reduces the ability to maintain PEEP in the 'good' lung, thus reducing alveolar recruitment resulting in worsening hypoxaemia.

SCC pp 91–96

A **48.** **A.** false **B.** true **C.** true **D.** false **E.** false

In open pneumothorax, caused by a penetrating injury, the lung on the affected side collapses and does not contribute to ventilation. Ventilation may be compromised in the healthy lung because of air exchange between the two lungs, mediastinal shift towards the good lung and because of inadequate expansion due to the weight of the affected collapsed lung. There is usually tachypnoea and respiratory distress.

SCC p 95

A **49.** **A.** true **B.** true **C.** false **D.** true **E.** false

In tension pneumothorax air enters the pleural space with ventilation and is unable to escape, usually due to a tissue fragment acting as a one way valve at the site of injury. The intrapleural pressure on the affected side becomes positive and may increase to over 40 mmHg. The increased intrapleural pressure 'pushes' the mediastinum towards the side of the healthy lung so reducing effective ventilation. The trachea will be deviated away from the collapsed lung. Tension pneumothorax is a medical emergency and the diagnosis is clinical. The risk of cardio-respiratory compromise or arrest is significant, and action needs to be immediate. There should be no delay for CXR.

SCC p 53, p 95

A **50.** **A.** true **B.** false **C.** false **D.** false **E.** true

CO_2 is converted to HCO_3^- and H^+ by carbonic anhydrase, and over 80% is carried in this way. Most of the HCO_3^- formed diffuses out of the red blood cell (RBC) into the plasma. To maintain electrical neutrality Cl^- ions diffuse from the plasma into the RBC (chloride shift). Carbamino compounds are mainly formed with haemoglobin, with less than a tenth being combined with plasma proteins. A small amount of CO_2 is transported dissolved in plasma despite its greater affinity than O_2.

SCC pp 66–69

A **51.** **A.** false **B.** false **C.** true **D.** false **E.** false

Haemoglobin is the principle buffer of H^+ liberated by the transport of CO_2. The binding (buffering) capacity of deoxyhaemoglobin is higher than oxyhaemoglobin which is manifest by the lower pH (i.e. more H^+ ions transported) of venous blood. By buffering the liberated H^+ ions from the reaction:

$$CO_2 + H_2O \rightleftharpoons HCO_3^- + H^+$$

More CO_2 can be taken up in the blood for transport. This is the Haldane effect. Chloride shift refers to intracellular (RBC) movement of Cl^- therefore venous blood RBC have more Cl^- than arterial.

SCC pp 66–69

A 52. **A.** false **B.** false **C.** true **D.** true **E.** false

Haemoglobin is a protein of 65,000 Daltons. Haem is a complex of porphyrin and Fe^{2+}. As O_2 combines with the haem groups the affinity for the remaining groups increases, hence the sigmoid shape of the curve. The oxygen carrying capacity of the blood is determined by the following formula:

$$O_2 \text{ capacity} = (Hb \times {}^{Sat}\!/_{100} \times 1.34) + (PaO_2 \times 0.003)$$

1.34 is a constant (the number of millilitres carried by 1 g Hb). It can be seen that by far the most significant factor in oxygen carrying capacity is the Hb × sat. By increasing full saturated Hb the O_2 content is increased most significantly. The dissolved portion is relatively minor and unimportant.

SCC pp 66–69

A 53. **A.** true **B.** false **C.** false **D.** true **E.** false

A left shift increases the slope of the oxyhaemoglobin dissociation curve (ODC) because of the increased affinity of Hb for O_2. Conversely a right shift decreases the affinity of Hb for O_2, and the O_2 is more easily released to the tissues. The Bohr effect refers to the shift to the right of the ODC caused by increased levels of CO_2 in the tissues. This allows oxygen to be liberated since the affinity of Hb for O_2 is reduced. The ODC is moved to the right by ↑ CO_2 (Bohr effect), ↑ temp and ↑ 2,3-diphosphoglycerate (2,3-DPG). 2,3-DPG binds avidly to deoxyhaemoglobin.

A **54.** **A.** false   **B.** false   **C.** true   **D.** false   **E.** true

Mixed venous saturation corresponds to P75 and is usually
5.3 kPa. P50 represents the level at which Hb is 50% loaded with
O_2 and is usually 3.46 kPa. P50 is used as an index of right or left
shift of the ODC. Left shift increases P50 and conversely right
shift decreases. Fetal Hb, myoglobin and CO dissociation curves
all lie to the left of the ODC. Fetal Hb has a higher affinity for O_2
than adult Hb and therefore retains O_2 at low PaO_2.
Methaemoglobin has a flat dissociation curve and is formed
when ferrous iron is oxidised to ferric. Methaemoglobin has no
affinity for O_2.

A **55.** **A.** false   **B.** false   **C.** false   **D.** false   **E.** true

Hyperoxia may develop because of increased inspired
concentration or increased total pressure of O_2, as occurs during
diving. The critical level for O_2 toxicity is 40 kPa and the risks
increase as the P_IO_2 increases, and with prolonged exposure.
Lung damage occurs due to decreased surfactant production and
resultant absorption atelectasis and airway collapse. Initial
symptoms are coughing and pain during breathing, this can lead
to convulsions and loss of consciousness. Infants are more
susceptible to oxygen toxicity and may be rendered blind if
exposed to $P_IO_2 > 40$ kPa due to damage to vitreous body.

SCC pp 76–78

A **56.** **A.** true   **B.** false   **C.** false   **D.** false   **E.** true

Surface tension exists in the lungs at the boundary of between
liquid and gas in the alveoli. Laplace's law states that the wall
tension is directly proportional to the product of transmural
pressure and cylinder radius. Because of this relationship alveoli
of smaller diameter experience higher surface tension forces and
would tend to empty into a larger alveolus. Surfactant lowers
surface tension and is more effective in smaller alveoli. Surfactant
deficiency leads to airway collapse. This may be seen in
premature infants who have reduced levels of surfactant, leading
to respiratory distress syndrome (RDS).

SCC pp 59–60

A 57. **A.** false **B.** false **C.** true **D.** false **E.** false

Dead space can be divided into anatomical, corresponding to the conducting airways down to the terminal bronchioles; and alveolar dead space. These together form physiological dead space. Anatomical dead space is measured by Fowler's nitrogen washout method. Physiological dead space is measured using the Bohr equation and is often fractionally larger than anatomical dead space because it takes account of under proposed alveoli. Anatomical dead space is usually of the order of 2 ml/kg or 150 ml for an average adult. Dead space accounts for about a third of tidal volume.

SCC pp 59–60

A 1. **A.** false   **B.** true   **C.** false   **D.** false   **E.** true

Glasgow (& Ranson's) criteria are used for indication of a severe attack of pancreatitis. The defined criteria are:

- Age > 55 years
- White cell count (WCC) > 15 × 10⁹/l
- Urea > 16 mmol/l
- Glucose > 10 mmol/l
- Calcium < 2 mmol/l
- Albumin < 32 g/l
- Arterial pO_2 < 8kPa
- Lactate dehydrogenase (LDH) > 600 iu/l

Surgery 1999 17: 11; 261–265   SCC pp 131–135

A 2. **A.** true   **B.** false   **C.** true   **D.** false   **E.** true

The following are factors influencing rebleeding:

- Age > 60
- Shock on admission
- Chronic rather than acute ulcer
- Gastric ulcer
- Underlying medical problem
- Bleeding source unknown
- >5 unit transfusion
- Bleeding from varices or malignancy

Surgery 1999 17: 12; 293–298   SCC pp 129–131

A 3. **A.** false   **B.** false   **C.** false   **D.** false   **E.** true

Organ failure in severe pancreatitis is usually respiratory, cardiovascular, renal then disseminated intravascular coagulation (DIC). Two organ system failure has a mortality of about 55% whereas three or more is associated with a mortality of >90%.

Hypercalcaemia and hypomagnesaemia are the most common metabolic disturbances and solid infected necrosis requires surgical debridement. Positive end expiratory pressure (PEEP) may prevent the development of adult respiratory distress syndrome (ARDS).

Surgery 1999 17: 11; 261–265   SCC pp 131–135

A 4.   A. true   **B.** false   **C.** false   **D.** true   **E.** false

Vesical distension is common, supravesical uncommon.
A percutaneous nephrostomy should be performed to decompress a supravesical obstruction. For pelvic malignancy, double J stents should be used palliatively and nephrostomy tubes avoided.

Surgery 1996 14: 12; 272–275   SCC pp 117–124

A 5.   A. true   **B.** false   **C.** true   **D.** false   **E.** false

Most chest injuries can be managed by intercostal tube drainage, analgesia and appropriate fluid management. Massive haemothorax is >1500 ml blood and blood loss of >200 ml is an indication for thoracotomy.

Surgery 1996 14: 1; 9–12   SCC pp 146–151

A 6.   A. true   **B.** true   **C.** true   **D.** true   **E.** true

Transected aorta is a typical high velocity deceleration injury. Bilateral rib fractures occur in major crush injuries.

Surgery 1996 14: 1; 9–12   SCC pp 146–151

A 7.   A. true   **B.** true   **C.** true   **D.** true   **E.** true

Hypovolaemia, decreased cardiac output haemorrhage, cardiac tamponade, pulmonary contusion, ventilatory failure and mediastinal disruption can all cause hypoxia following thoracic trauma.

Surgery 1996 14: 1; 9–12   SCC pp 146–151

A 8.   A. true   **B.** false   **C.** false   **D.** true   **E.** false

SCC pp 117–122

A 9. **A.** true **B.** true **C.** true **D.** true **E.** false

Extradural haematomas are associated with lucid intervals rather than subdural haematomas.

SCC pp 99–107

A 10. **A.** true **B.** false **C.** false **D.** false **E.** true

Features are:

Hypovolaemic shock	Tachycardia and hypotension
Neurogenic shock	Paralysis, bradycardia and hypotension
Spinal shock	Flaccid muscles, absent reflexes and loss of sensation

SCC pp 108–112

A 11. **A.** true **B.** false **C.** false **D.** true **E.** false

High flow oxygen therapy is necessary until carboxyhaemoglobin (COHb) levels are less than 10%. Smoke only causes damage to the larynx and pharynx. Early intubation should be performed if there are any doubts as to the airway.

SCC pp 151–157

A 12. **A.** false **B.** false **C.** false **D.** false **E.** false

Gastrointestinal stress ulceration is common. Virtually all critically ill patients have endoscopic evidence of it. Significant bleeds occur in 10–20%. In only 1–2% of cases does prophylaxis have any effect on mortality and outcome. H_2 antagonists should be used for high-risk patients. Surgical intervention is rarely necessary.

SCC pp 129–131

A 13. **A.** true **B.** false **C.** false **D.** true **E.** true

Inflammatory bowel disease and dysphagia are indications. Proximal small bowel fistulae, severe diarrhoea and small bowel obstruction are contra-indications as are ileus with dilated small intestine and severe pancreatitis.

SCC pp 140–146

A **14.** **A.** true **B.** false **C.** false **D.** true **E.** true

Daily full blood count (FBC), urea and electrolytes (U & E), glucose and prothrombin time.

Albumin is necessary twice weekly and calcium weekly.

SCC pp 140–146

A **15.** **A.** false **B.** false **C.** true **D.** false **E.** true

Rectal examination in patients with pelvic injury/fracture is mandatory to exclude open fractures or high riding prostate. Catheterisation should occur after urethral injury has been excluded. Airway, Breathing and Circulation (ABC) remains the priority.

SCC pp 146–151

A **16.** **A.** false **B.** false **C.** true **D.** true **E.** true

Hyperthermia is defined as a core temperature above 40.5°C and is associated with respiratory alkalosis. Dantrolene is used along with oxygen and the cessation of the anaesthetic to treat malignant hyperpyrexia.

A **17.** **A.** false **B.** true **C.** true **D.** false **E.** true

Leaks occur in 10–15% of colonic anastamoses. Dehydrated and shocked patients have a higher incidence of leaks. Percutaneous CT (or ultrasound) guided drainage may be useful.

A **18.** **A.** false **B.** false **C.** true **D.** false **E.** true

Cefuroxime is a 2nd generation cephalosporin. Penicillin/cephalosporin cross-hypersensitivity has an incidence of approximately 5–10%. They are both eliminated via the kidney.

SCC p 174

A **19.** **A.** true **B.** false **C.** true **D.** true **E.** false

The criteria are:

■ Haemodynamically stable after resuscitation
■ No persistent or increasing abdominal pain or tenderness

- No other peritoneal injuries requiring laparotomy
- <4 units blood transfusion required

Computerised tomography findings

- Haemoperitoneum <500 ml
- Simple hepatic parenchymal laceration or intra-hepatic haematoma

SCC pp 146–151

A 20. A. true   **B.** true   **C.** true   **D.** true   **E.** true

Peritonitis, evisceration and abdominal gunshot wounds are all indications for laparotomy as are uncontrolled haemorrhage, persistent shock and a clinical deterioration.

SCC pp 146–151

A 21. A. true   **B.** false   **C.** true   **D.** true   **E.** false

The commonest four complications are:

- Rebleeding (consider angiography and selective embolisation)
- Bile leaks (ERCP plus endoscopic sphincterotomy plus stenting)
- Ischaemic segments
- Infected fluid collections

CT/ultrasound can allow identification of collections and percutaneous drainage. Subhepatic sepsis (1 in 5 cases) usually relates to bile leak, ischaemic tissue, undrained collections or bowel injury.

A 22. A. false   **B.** false   **C.** false   **D.** true   **E.** true

Mortality after hepatic injury

- Overall 10–15%
- Penetrating (civilian) 1%
- Blunt > 20%
- Blunt (liver only) 10%
- Blunt (3 major organs injured) > 70%

Bleeding causes >50% of deaths.

SCC pp 146–151

A 23. A. true   **B.** true   **C.** false   **D.** false   **E.** true

A high index of suspicion is necessary to recognise pancreatic trauma. Abdominal X-ray (AXR) may show retroperitoneal air or diaphragmatic rupture. Serum amylase is a poor indicator and can be normal in patients with severe pancreatic damage. Contrast enhanced CT is the best investigation and demonstrates pancreatic oedema or swelling and collections. ERCP should be used to assess the ducts.

SCC pp 146–151

A 24. A. true   **B.** true   **C.** true   **D.** true   **E.** true

Pancreatic trauma can lead to pseudocyst, fistulae, ascites intra-abdominal abscess, wound infection, pancreatic abscess and acute and chronic pancreatitis.

SCC pp 146–151

A 25. A. true   **B.** false   **C.** true   **D.** true   **E.** true

Patients are usually managed on ITU. Enteral feeding recommences as early as possible. Daily LFTs are performed. Steroids are rapidly tailed off. Immunosuppressive regimes mostly include cyclosporin or tacrolimus with azathioprine, mycophenolate mofetil and prednisolone. Acute rejection occurs in 50% but is treated by extra steroids or an altered drug regimen. Infection is a major cause of morbidity.

SCC pp 135–139

A 26. A. false   **B.** true   **C.** true   **D.** false   **E.** true

Hepatocellular carcinoma has a low incidence of recurrence and as such a small tumour is not a contra-indication. Inability to comply with drug therapy is an additional contra-indication. Neuroendocrine tumours and sarcomata with liver metastases can do well with transplantation for several years.

SCC pp 135–139

A 27. A. true   **B.** true   **C.** true   **D.** false   **E.** false

The mortality if two other organ systems are involved is 95%. The electrolyte sequelae of acute renal failure (ARF) are hypocalcaemia, hyperkalaemia and metabolic acidosis. Uraemia can lead to pericarditis, drowsiness tremor and confusion.

Surgery 2000 18: 6; 135–138   `SCC` pp 117–122

A 28. **A.** true   **B.** true   **C.** true   **D.** true   **E.** true

Postoperative hepatic dysfunction may be due to excess bilirubin (transfusion or haemolysis), hepatocellular damage (pre-existing, viral hepatitis, sepsis, hypotension, hypoxaemia or halothane-induced hepatic necrosis) or extrahepatic biliary obstruction (gallstones, ascending cholangitis, pancreatitis or surgical damage to the common bile duct).

Surgery 2000 18: 7; 180–181   `SCC` pp 135–139

A 29. **A.** true   **B.** false   **C.** true   **D.** true   **E.** false

Platelet activating factor (PAF), TNF-α, Interleukins 1, 6, 8, 2, 10 and monocyte chemotactic protein-1 are the major inflammatory mediators in SIRS.

`SCC` pp 112–116

A 30. **A.** true   **B.** false   **C.** false   **D.** true   **E.** true

Major trauma results in increased prolactin, anti-diuretic hormone (ADH), catecholamine and cortisol and decreased thyroxine (T3 and T4).

`SCC` pp 146–151

A 31. **A.** true   **B.** true   **C.** true   **D.** true   **E.** true

Dose modification may be necessary with all antibiotics in patients with acute renal failure. Close monitoring is necessary.

`SCC` pp 117–122

A 32. **A.** true   **B.** true   **C.** true   **D.** true   **E.** true

Acute subdural injuries are associated with a lucid interval in approximately 10–15% of cases.

`SCC` pp 99–107

A 33. **A.** true   **B.** true   **C.** true   **D.** true   **E.** true

SCC pp 146–151

A 34. **A.** true   **B.** false   **C.** true   **D.** false   **E.** true

Burns patients require energy dense feeds but do not tolerate high volumes. 2000 ml feeds provide 70 g protein typically. Glutamine is an essential amino acid.

SCC pp 140–146

A 35. **A.** true   **B.** false   **C.** true   **D.** true   **E.** true

Complications are:

Mechanical	tube blockage, aspiration, naso-pharyngeal irritation, tube misplacement
Infection	occurs more with parenteral nutrition
Physiological	diarrhoea, hypoalbuminaemia, nausea and vomiting, hyperglycaemia, hypercapnia, fluid overload

SCC pp 140–146

A 36. **A.** false   **B.** false   **C.** false   **D.** false   **E.** false

Haemothorax is the commonest injury and 80% require nothing more than an intercostal chest drain.

SCC pp 146–151

A 37. **A.** true   **B.** false   **C.** true   **D.** false   **E.** true

Epidural haematoma classically have a lucid interval (although subdural haemotoma (SDH) have one in about 15%) and carry the better prognosis. Intra-cranial pressure (ICP) in an adult should be less than 15 mmHg. Management is geared at the prevention of secondary brain injury and involves oxygenation and ventilation and the maintenance of cerebral perfusion pressure (CPP) >60 mmHg.

SCC pp 99–107

A. true   **B.** false   **C.** true   **D.** true   **E.** true

ICP requires treatment at levels >15 mmHg. Sedation decreases cerebral blood flow. Aggressive hyperventilation can increase ICP.

SCC pp 99–107

A 39. **A.** true   **B.** true   **C.** true   **D.** true   **E.** true

Monitoring of pressure areas should also be performed.

SCC pp 108–112

A 40. **A.** true   **B.** true   **C.** false   **D.** false   **E.** true

Pulmonary sepsis is the leading cause of death.
The hypermetabolic response peaks at 7–10 days.

SCC pp 151–157

A 41. **A.** false   **B.** true   **C.** true   **D.** true   **E.** true

Respiratory insufficiency forms part of a failure to respond to ICU therapy.

SCC pp 131–135

A 42. **A.** true   **B.** true   **C.** false   **D.** false   **E.** false

Fractional excretion Na < 1%; urine Cr/plasma Cr > 40 are suggestive of pre-renal renal failure.

Other features include urinary blood urea nitrogen (BUN)/plasma BUN > 8; plasma BUN/Cr > 20, urine sodium < 20 mmol/L and urine osmolality > 500 mosm/kg H_2O.

SCC pp 117–122

A 43. **A.** true   **B.** false   **C.** true   **D.** false   **E.** true

95% of potassium is intracellular. Hartmann's solution should be avoided in renal failure as it contains potassium and can lead to hyperkalaemia. The stress response to surgery also results in water retention.

SCC p 140

A 44. **A.** false **B.** false **C.** true **D.** false **E.** false

Fat embolism most commonly occurs after long bone fracture. Reaming and the insertion of intramedullary nails also increase risk. Heparinisation is not only unnecessary but may lead to compartment syndrome. High dependency/intensive care monitoring is essential and ventilation may be necessary. Development of fat embolism syndrome (FES) occurs in approximately 5%. Fat embolism is rare in pancreatitis.

SCC pp 158–160

A 45. **A.** true **B.** false **C.** false **D.** true **E.** true

Symptoms and signs of FES:

- Respiratory – dyspnoea, tachypnoea, hypoxaemia, ARDS, infiltrates on CXR
- CNS – anxiety, irritation, confusion, convulsions, cerebral oedema on CT
- Other – petechial rash, retinal haemorrhages, tachycardia, fever

SCC pp 158–160

A 46. **A.** true **B.** true **C.** true **D.** true **E.** true

Blood loss is mediated by hypovolaemic shock.

SCC pp 146–151

A 47. **A.** true **B.** false **C.** true **D.** false **E.** false

SCC pp 135–139

A 48. **A.** true **B.** true **C.** true **D.** true **E.** false

Age has no effect on the risk of developing ATN.

SCC pp 117–122

A 49. **A.** true **B.** false **C.** true **D.** true **E.** false

Benzyl penicillin may cause nephritis.

SCC pp 117–122

A 50. **A.** true   **B.** true   **C.** true   **D.** true   **E.** true

Table 3.1 Criteria for transfer to a burns centre

Second- and third-degree burns >10% TBSA in patients <10 or >50 years of age

Second- and third-degree burns to >20% TBSA in all other ages

Third-degree burns >5% TBSA in patients of any age

All second- and third-degree burns with the threat of functional or cosmetic impairment to the face, hands, feet, genitalia, perineum or major joints

All electrical burns, including lightning injuries

Chemical burns

Burns involving inhalation injury

Circumferential burns of the extremities and/or chest

Burns involving concomitant trauma among which the burn injury poses the greatest risk of morbidity or mortality.

Burns in patients with pre-existing medical conditions that may complicate management and/or prolong recovery, such as coronary artery disease, lung disease or diabetes.

SCC pp 151–157

A 51. **A.** false   **B.** true   **C.** true   **D.** true   **E.** false

Metabolic acidosis may be classified into those with a normal or high anion gap. The normal cations present in plasma are Na, K, Ca, Mg. The normal anions are Cl, HCO_3, and negative charges present on albumin, phosphate, sulphate, lactate, and other organic acids. The sum of negative and positive charges must be equal. The readily measured cations and anions give the anion gap according to the equation:

$$\text{Anion gap} = \{[Na] + [K]\} - \{[Cl] + [HCO_3]\}$$

Because there are more unmeasured anions than cations, the normal anion gap is 10–18 mmol/l. Lactic acidosis is characterised by a high anion gap because the unmeasured lactate anion is present in increased quantities.

Increased lactic acid production occurs when cellular respiration is abnormal (type A) or due to a metabolic abnormality (type B). The commonest cause of lactic acidosis is poor tissue perfusion due to cardiogenic shock, post cardiac arrest, or sepsis (type A).

Type B lactic acidosis may be caused by liver failure or metformin accumulation, typically in renal failure.

The management of lactic acidosis should address the underlying cause and aims to optimise tissue perfusion and oxygen delivery through volume replacement, ventilatory and inotropic support. The administration of sodium bicarbonate may theoretically worsen intracellular acidosis through increased generation of CO_2 and should be limited to severe acidosis (e.g. pH < 7.1).

A 52. A. false **B.** true **C.** true **D.** false **E.** true

DIC is characterised by activation of the clotting cascades with generation of fibrin, consumption of clotting factors and platelets, and secondary activation of fibrinolysis leading to production of fibrinogen degradation products (FDPs). DIC may be asymptomatic manifest only on blood investigations, or may result in bleeding, or tissue ischaemia due to vessel occlusion by fibrin and platelets.

The prothrombin time (or international normalised ratio (INR)), activated partial thromboplastin time (APTT), and thrombin time are usually prolonged. The fibrinogen level and platelet count are low. High levels of FDPs are present. There may be fragmented red cells on the blood film due to red cell damage during passage through fibrin webs in the circulation. Treatment is aimed at correcting the underlying cause. Blood product support (platelets, fresh frozen plasma (FFP), cryoprecipitate, packed red cells) is given under haematology advice.

SCC pp 47–49

A 53. A. true **B.** false **C.** true **D.** false **E.** true

DIC may be caused by gram-negative, meningococcal and staphylococcal septicaemia, tissue damage after trauma, burns or surgery, malignancy, haemolytic blood transfusion reactions, falciparum malaria, snake bites, and obstetric conditions such as placental abruption and amniotic fluid embolism.

SCC pp 47–49

A 54. A. false **B.** false **C.** true **D.** true **E.** true

These arterial blood gases demonstrate an acidosis (the pH is <7.36). Respiratory acidosis is caused by retention of CO_2, most commonly due to chronic obstructive pulmonary disease (COPD), so this case cannot be respiratory in origin because the pCO_2 is low. The primary abnormality must be the low bicarbonate either due to increased bicarbonate loss, or more commonly due to its consumption to buffer increased acid production or reduced acid excretion. This is therefore a metabolic acidosis, and the pCO_2 is low as the patient hyperventilates to blow off CO_2. This is called respiratory compensation for metabolic acidosis. Respiratory failure is not present because there is neither hypoxia or hypercapnoea.

Metabolic acidosis may be caused by:

■ Failure to excrete acid, e.g. renal failure, type I (distal) and type IV renal tubular acidosis
■ Ingestion of acid, e.g. salicylate poisoning
■ Excess production of acid, e.g. diabetic ketoacidosis
■ Anaerobic production of lactic acid
■ Increased production of hydrochloric acid (high protein intake)
■ Increased bicarbonate loss, e.g. gastrointestinal from diarrhoea, ileostomy, ureterosigmoidoscopy, or renal in type II (proximal) renal tubular acidosis

SCC pp 112–122

A 55. A. false **B.** false **C.** true **D.** true **E.** true

These arterial blood gases demonstrate type II respiratory failure. Respiratory failure is classified into type I, in which pCO_2 is normal or low, and type II in which pCO_2 is elevated, as in this case. Causes of type I respiratory failure include COPD, pulmonary oedema, pneumonia, ARDS, pulmonary embolism and fibrosing alveolitis. Type II respiratory failure may be caused by COPD, depression of the respiratory centre (e.g. opiates, benzodiazepines), respiratory muscle weakness, and chest wall deformities.

There is also a respiratory acidosis: the pH is low indicating acidosis, and the pCO_2 is raised indicating that CO_2 retention is the cause of the acidosis. In chronic respiratory acidosis (most commonly caused by COPD), renal retention of bicarbonate is increased. This is known as metabolic compensation. In this case, the bicarbonate concentration is normal, suggesting that the respiratory acidosis is acute. Severe acute asthma initially results in hyperventilation with a low pCO_2. In a life-threatening attack, the pCO_2 may rise as the patient tires. This is a grave sign and is an indication for mechanical ventilation.

SCC pp 79–80

A 56. A. true **B.** true **C.** false **D.** false **E.** false

Systemic inflammatory response syndrome (SIRS) is a protective inflammatory response to an insult or invading pathogen. Tissue injury acts as a precipitant and the common causes are infection, trauma, tumour invasion, hypoxia and ischaemia. Burns patients are particularly susceptible to SIRS which is a considerable cause of morbidity. The immune reaction is not abnormal but paradoxically leads to further tissue damage because of hypovolaemia and resultant poor tissue perfusion. Although multi-organ dysfunction syndrome (MODS) is a consequence of SIRS, the progression is not automatic and can be avoided by clinical intervention.

SCC pp 112–116

A 57. A. false **B.** true **C.** true **D.** true **E.** true

The diagnosis of SIRS is made by the patient fulfilling two or more of the following criteria:

I.   Core temperature > 38 or <36°C
II. Heart rate > 90 beats per minute
III. Respiratory rate > 20 breaths per minute or $PaCO_2$ < 4.26 kPa
IV. WCC > 12 $\times$ 10^9/l or <4 $\times$ 10^9 (with >10% neutrophils or immature forms)

SCC pp 112–116

A 58. A. true **B.** false **C.** false **D.** false **E.** true

Typically the patient will have warm, flushed peripheries, with diastolic hypotension and tachycardia. Nitric oxide exerts a relaxant effect on the vasculature, opposing the myogenic contraction of the vessel walls. Metabolic acidosis may occur as a result of tissue hypoperfusion and lactic acid formation. The patient may have deranged clotting function, because of activation of the coagulation cascade, with the clotting factors being consumed in the reaction. This is also referred to as consumptive coagulopathy.

SCC pp 112–116

A 59. **A.** false   **B.** false   **C.** true   **D.** false   **E.** true

MODS is a progression from SIRS diagnosed by dysfunction of two or more organ systems. The inflammatory process of SIRS results in hypoperfusion and tissue ischaemia. There is interstitial oedema from extravasation of fluid from damaged vascular endothelium. Oliguria occurs due to hypovolaemia and hypoperfusion and occurs relatively early, often during SIRS. If treated promptly this can be reversible and not a sign of end organ damage. As hypoperfusion continues, renal dysfunction becomes more difficult to reverse and treat. With prompt treatment with fluid resuscitation and other supportive measures progression to irreversible multi-organ failure syndrome (MOFS) can be avoided.

SCC pp 112–116

A 60. **A.** false   **B.** false   **C.** false   **D.** false   **E.** false

Fluid therapy is essential to counteract tissue hypoperfusion from hypovolaemia. Careful monitoring is required however, since there is a risk of worsening tissue oedema. With acute lung injury, the risk of worsening respiratory function is increased with inappropriate use of large volumes of fluids. Fluid resuscitation is key to prevention of deteriorating organ function but must be balanced with appropriate use of inotropes. Inotropes which increase afterload (α agonists) are often required but can cause myocardial dysfunction. β agonists are used to treat myocardial dysfunction and to maintain tissue perfusion. Measurement of cardiac output is desirable but not mandatory since invasive methods do carry a risk of morbidity, particularly if there is coagulopathy. Arterial monitoring is not contra-indicated since the risk of distal ischaemia is small and it provides essential information for prescribing inotropes.

SCC pp 112–116

A 61. A. false **B.** true **C.** false **D.** true **E.** false

The mortality rate depends on the number of organ systems affected and the duration of failure:

Number of failed organ systems	Mortality rate on day 1	Mortality rate on day 4
2	50%	65%
3	80%	95%

Mortality is higher at extremes of age, with the presence of sepsis, burns and immunocompromise. The pre-morbid health of the patient is also important in outcome.

SCC pp 112–116

A 62. A. true **B.** true **C.** false **D.** false **E.** true

Intracellular K^+ is usually 155 mmol/l, and is the most concentrated intracellular ion. Sodium is the most abundant extracellular ion. The daily Ca^{2+} requirement is 0.17 mmol/kg/day. Mg^{2+} is mainly intracellular with a concentration of 2 mmol/l.

SCC p 140

A 63. A. false **B.** false **C.** true **D.** true **E.** false

5% dextrose has an osmolality of 278 mosmol/kg which is less than that of blood at 290 mosmol/kg. Hartmann's solution has a Na^+ concentration of 131 mmol/l and Cl^- concentration of 111 mmol/l. Both N/saline and Hartmann's solution are slightly hypertonic compared to blood, and are distributed in the ECF. D/saline is distributed equally between ICF and ECF. 5% dextrose is distributed throughout total body water.

SCC p 140

A 64. A. true **B.** false **C.** false **D.** true **E.** true

As a general rule replace like with like. Peritonitis results in a loss of protein rich exudate and potentially large fluid shifts.

Replacement should be with a fluid with high colloid osmotic pressure. Albumin or artificial colloids could also be used. Loss of ECF volume by vomiting or diarrhoea should be replaced by N/saline or Hartmann's solution. Diabetes mellitus tends to lose ECF by polyuria, Hartmann's solution contains lactate, so increasing the risk of lactic acidosis. N/saline should be used. Diabetes insipidus loses total body water and should be replaced by water (or 5% dextrose). Care should be taken with 5% dextrose however if there is a co-existing head injury since cerebral oedema may be precipitated. Burns may cause bleeding from the initial insult or after theatre debridement. Any colloid may be used but if blood is lost it should be replaced.

`SCC` p 140

A **65.** **A.** false   **B.** false   **C.** true   **D.** false   **E.** true

Body mass index is weight/height^2

- Normal value is 20–25
- 25–30 is over weight
- 30–35 is obese
- >35 is morbidly obese

Energy requirements are 20–30 kcal/kg/day, usually 2000 kcal for females, 2500 kcal for males. Nitrogen requirement for females is 7.5 g/day. In non-catabolic patients 1 g N should be given for every 200 kcal energy.

`SCC` pp 140–146

A **66.** **A.** true   **B.** false   **C.** false   **D.** false   **E.** false

Nutrition should be modified in organ failure

- Respiratory
  - high fat, low carbohydrate (to limit CO_2 production)
- Renal
  - low nitrogen (to reduce urea production)
  - low fat (poor handling)
  - low sodium and water (to reduce fluid overload)
  - low potassium
- Cardiac
  - low sodium and water (to reduce fluid overload)

- Liver
  - low sodium and water
  - low nitrogen (in encephalopathic patients)
  - adequate carbohydrate load (since they tend towards hypoglycaemia)
- Cerebral
  - close blood glucose control required
  - glucose is the main substrate and hypoglycaemia should be avoided
  - hyperglycaemia will worsen cerebral oedema

SCC pp 140–146

A 67. A. false **B.** false **C.** true **D.** false **E.** false

Enteral feeding has a number of advantages over the parenteral route:

- Enteral feeding is more physiological and allows substrates to be absorbed more gradually into the bloodstream
- Gastric protection unnecessary since the feed lines the stomach (protects against stress ulceration)
- Maintains function of the gut and prevents atrophy reducing the risk of translocation of gut bacteria

Parenteral nutrition should only be used if enteral nutrition is not possible. There is no advantage to short term (days) use of parenteral nutrition. It will often lead to hyperglycaemia and increases insulin requirements. Bowel sounds are notoriously poor at predicting the function of the gut. Absence of bowel sounds does not mean that enteral nutrition should not be attempted.

SCC pp 140–146

A 68. A. true **B.** true **C.** true **D.** false **E.** false

Fats and carbohydrates are broken down to CO_2 and water, but proteins are only broken down as far as urea. Fat gives twice as much energy per gram than carbohydrate or protein. About 65% of the calories required per day comes from carbohydrate, 25% from fat and 15% from protein. A high protein diet increases the basal metabolic rate (BMR) since more energy is required to produce 1mol ATP from protein than carbohydrate (about 20%)

$$\text{Respiratory quotient (RQ)} = \frac{\dot{V}CO_2}{\dot{V}O_2} = \frac{\text{rate of } CO_2 \text{ formation}}{\text{rate of } O_2 \text{ uptake}}$$

RQ varies with diet, with carbohydrate the RQ is 1.0, for fats the RQ is 0.7. Since the proportion of protein in the diet varies relatively little the overall RQ will vary between 0.7 (fatty diet) and 1.0 (carbohydrate diet).

SCC pp 140–146

A 1. **A.** false **B.** false **C.** false **D.** true **E.** true

Diagnosis of brainstem death (BSD) in the UK.

Preconditions:

- Diagnosis compatible with BSD
- Presence of irreversible structural brain damage
- Presence of apnoeic coma

Exclusions:

- Drugs, Hypothermia, Metabolic abnormalities, Intoxication

Clinical Tests:

- Absent brain stem reflexes
  — No pupil response to light
  — No corneal reflex
  — No gag reflex
  — No cough reflex
  — No vestibulo-ocular reflex (50 ml ice-cold water)
- Persistant apnoea

Surgery 1999 17: 9; 205–207   SCC pp 183–185

A 2. **A.** true **B.** false **C.** true **D.** false **E.** false

Deep infections with implants can occur more than a year after surgery.

Operative wound infection rates:

- Clean 0.8%
- Clean-contaminated 1.3%
- Contaminated 10.2%

Latex and silastic drains increase the rate of infection following abdominal surgery.

Wounds should be shaved (or preferably clipped) immediately prior to surgery.

Surgery 1999 17: 6; 126–130　　　　　　　SCC pp 175–179

A 3. **A.** false **B.** false **C.** false **D.** true **E.** false

Fat embolism syndrome (FES) occurs in approximately 5% of cases. FES is rarely seen with pancreatitis but does occur. Crush injuries cause fat embolism more than open injuries. Fat embolism results in hypoxaemia and hypocarbia on ABG analysis.

SCC pp 158–160

A 4. **A.** true **B.** false **C.** false **D.** true **E.** true

Respiratory signs of FES are dyspnoea, tachypnoea, hypoxaemia, bilateral infiltrates on CXR and ARDS. CNS signs include anxiety, irritation, confusion, convulsions and cerebral oedema on CT. Other signs are a petechial rash, retinal haemorrhages, tachycardia and fever. Laboratory tests include sudden anaemia and thrombocytopenia and a raised ESR.

SCC pp 158–160

A 5. **A.** true **B.** true **C.** false **D.** false **E.** false

Age	Heart rate (HR)	Blood pressure (systolic)	Respiratory rate (RR)
<1 year	120–140	70–90	30–40
2–5 years	100–120	80–90	20–30
5–12 years	80–120	90–110	15–20

A 6. **A.** false **B.** false **C.** true **D.** true **E.** false

Two sets of tests performed by two practitioners registered for more than 5 years, one of whom is a consultant, and neither of whom members of the transplant team are required.

Tests:

■ Pupils fixed and dilated
■ No corneal reflex

- No vestibulo-ocular reflexes
- No CNS motor responses
- No gag reflex
- No respiratory effort

SCC pp 183–185

A 7. **A.** true **B.** true **C.** true **D.** false **E.** false

Diabetes is a risk for oropharyngeal colonisation but not nosocomial pneumonia.

SCC pp 165–166, pp 175–177

A 8. **A.** true **B.** true **C.** false **D.** false **E.** false

Head injury – *Staphylococcus aureus*
Ventilation – *Pseudomonas*
Thoracoabdominal surgery – anaerobes
Tracheotomy – *Pseudomonas*

SCC pp 175–177

A 9. **A.** true **B.** true **C.** true **D.** true **E.** true

As always – culture and seek microbiological advice – and appropriate 'best guess' antibiotics. The suggested antibiotics may not be the best, but they are appropriate.

SCC pp 175–177

A 1. **A.** true   **B.** false   **C.** false   **D.** false   **E.** true

The acute physiology and chronic health evaluation (APACHE) score is the most commonly used scoring system in intensive therapy unit (ITU).

SCC pp 198–201

A 2. **A.** true   **B.** true   **C.** false   **D.** false   **E.** false

Diamorphine is metabolised by ester hydrolysis in the liver, plasma and central nervous system (CNS). Its half life is 5 minutes and it is less of a respiratory depressant than morphine. It may be given safely intrathecally.

SCC pp 203–205

A 3. **A.** false   **B.** true   **C.** true   **D.** false   **E.** true

Epidural opioids are 10 times more potent than intravenous. Epidural haematoma may lead to cord compression and urinary retention occurs in 30%.

Surgery 2000 18: 8; 198–201   SCC pp 203–205

A 4. **A.** true   **B.** false   **C.** true   **D.** true   **E.** true

See early warning table in Viva Answers, p 226.

SCC pp 189–191

A 5. **A.** true   **B.** true   **C.** true   **D.** true   **E.** true

Early diagnosis and prompt treatment improves outcome, increased age, illness severity and decreased physiological reserve are all detrimental.

SCC pp 198–201

A 6.   **A.** false   **B.** true   **C.** false   **D.** true   **E.** true

Alfentanil is not sedative. Fentanyl unlike morphine does not cause histamine release.

SCC pp 203–205

A 7.   **A.** true   **B.** false   **C.** false   **D.** false   **E.** true

Median nerve neuropathy can arise from a haematoma following a brachial artery catheter. Up to 50% of radial artery catheters are associated with Doppler proven intra-arterial thromboses. A maximum rate of 6% for pneumothoraces after central line insertion has been demonstrated. Thoracic duct injury usually resolves with compression.

SCC pp 205–207

A 8.   **A.** false   **B.** false   **C.** false   **D.** true   **E.** true

The aim of scoring systems used clinically is to evaluate outcome for different groups of intensive care unit (ICU) patients. Scoring systems, do not predict outcome or guide treatment planning for individual patients. They may be used to determine patient groups according to severity of illness, attach risk to different groups or compare patient groups in ICU's from different hospitals. Risk adjustment takes into account the differences between patients that affects their risk of a particular outcome e.g. age, premorbid illness, severity of illness or emergency surgery. These factors constitute the case-mix, case-mix adjustment is the process of accounting for these in the comparison of any outcome measure.

SCC pp 198–201

A 9.   **A.** false   **B.** false   **C.** false   **D.** true   **E.** true

The revised trauma score (RTS) correlates well with survival so that a high score is better. RTS12 is associated with 99.5% survival and RTS0 3.7% survival. The scores range from 0 to 12 by a combination of Glasgow coma score (GCS), systolic blood pressure and respiratory rate (RR).

SCC pp 198–201

A 10. **A.** false **B.** false **C.** true **D.** true **E.** false

APACHE stands for acute physiology and chronic health evaluation. None of these scoring systems provides any predictive power over individual treatment progression or outcome. They are designed to stratify patients into groups depending on the acute physiological insult and take into account some aspect of significant chronic medical problems.

SCC pp 198–201

A 11. **A.** false **B.** false **C.** true **D.** false **E.** true

The abbreviated injury score (AIS) is calculated by the sum of the squares of the three highest categories from the injury severity scale (ISS). From AIS the lethal dose in 50% (LD 50) has been calculated.

This is age dependent and is 40 for 15–44 years, 29 for 45–64 years and 20 for those >65 years. In ISS there are seven anatomical areas and loss of consciousness (LOC) for 12 minutes scores 2.

SCC pp 198–201

A 12. **A.** false **B.** true **C.** true **D.** false **E.** false

Thiopentone is a barbiturate compound which is metabolised in the liver. Thiopentone tends to accumulate with repeated doses and therefore is not suitable for prolonged use in general ICU patients. It is occasionally used by infusion on neuro ICU's to reduce the metabolic demand for oxygen of the damaged brain. Prolonged infusion requires electroencephalogram (EEG) monitoring. Propofol is an emulsion in soya fat and therefore has a high lipid content. Ketamine is not a conventional induction agent for anaesthesia because it does not have a clearly defined sleep point. It tends to be used as an analgesic and anaesthetic in field conditions e.g. military campaign. Midazolam is often used in long term infusion but it is metabolised in the liver to active drugs which have sedative properties. Drugs used in ICU for infusions should be stopped periodically in order to assess their effect on consciousness, to avoid prolonged coma.

SCC pp 203–205

A 13. **A.** true **B.** false **C.** true **D.** true **E.** false

Midazolam is a water soluble benzodiazepine which is used for sedation as infusion and bolus. It has a relatively short duration of action as a bolus but cumulates readily when given by infusion leading to prolonged coma. To prevent this patients should be assessed frequently and their sedation adjusted. Midazolam is popular by infusion because it is cheap, water soluble, can be given in relatively concentrated infusions and is reasonably familiar to use. One arm-brain circulation time is about 30 seconds and sedatives used for rapid sequence induction should have their effects within this.

SCC pp 203–205

A 14. **A.** true **B.** true **C.** true **D.** false **E.** false

Despite their similar elimination half lives of about 4 hours, morphine is longer acting because of the rapid redistribution of the more lipid soluble fentanyl. Alfentanil has the shortest duration of action of the commonly used sedatives on ICU. Fentanyl and Alfentanil infusions can continue for prolonged periods without precipitating prolonged coma. Morphine has two active metabolites which can cause prolonged sedation and apnoea. Morphine causes histamine release and should be used with care in asthmatic patients.

SCC pp 203–205

A 15. **A.** true **B.** false **C.** true **D.** false **E.** true

All opioids have the tendency to cause chest wall rigidity to some degree. Fentanyl and the new ultra-short acting opioid remifentanil seem to be more responsible than the others. All opioid effects are reversed by naloxone including respiratory depression, euphoria and nausea. Morphine 3 and 6 sulphate are both active metabolites and tend to accumulate with prolonged infusions. This is particularly true in patients with hepatic or renal failure where fentanyl or alfentanil would be a more sensible choice. All opioids cause some degree of vasodilatation by a central action, the amount of accompanying hypotension depends on the individual drug. Morphine tends to cause more hypotension than alfentanil or fentanyl.

SCC pp 203–205

A **16.** **A.** true **B.** false **C.** false **D.** false **E.** true

Rocuronium works within 60 seconds and can be used as an alternative to suxamethonium for rapid sequence intubation. Atracurium is an ester which is kept refrigerated because it undergoes spontaneous breakdown at room temperature, called Hoffmann degradation which is enzyme independent. Atracurium is the drug of choice for ICU infusions and in renal failure since it does not accumulate. Vecuronium is a steroid which is metabolised in the liver and should be avoided in hepatic failure because of the risk of accumulation and prolonged paralysis. Vecuronium has an onset of 2–3 minutes.

SCC pp 203–205

A **17.** **A.** true **B.** false **C.** false **D.** true **E.** false

Suxamethonium is a depolarising muscle relaxant which 'activates' the neuromuscular junction causing visible faciculation before temporarily paralysing it. It causes depolarisation because suxamethonium is structurally related to two acetyl choline molecules joined together, thereby activating the receptor. Suxamethonium is metabolised by plasma cholinesterase, an enzyme produced by the liver which acts locally. Suxamethonium has a number of side-effects including myalgia in young adults, hyperkalaemia in burns and spinal injury patients and raised intra-optic and intra-cranial pressure (these latter two are temporary). Suxamethonium has rapid onset and offset and is primarily used for rapid sequence intubation.

SCC pp 203–205

A **18.** **A.** false **B.** false **C.** true **D.** false **E.** false

Osmolarity is the concentration of a solution expressed as osmoles of solute per litre of solution (mosmol/l). Osmolality is the concentration of a solution expressed as osmoles of solute per kg solvent (mosmol/kg). Osmolality is independent of temperature and volume taken up by solutes within the solutions. Osmolality is the measure most often used clinically, and is estimated by depression of freezing point. Semipermeable membranes allow solvent (fluid) but not solute (particles) to pass through. The osmolality of plasma is 290 mosmol/kg H_2O.

SCC pp 117–122

A **19.** **A.** true **B.** false **C.** false **D.** false **E.** false

The kidney has a number of metabolic functions including gluconeogenesis, peptide hydrolysis and arginine formation. Each kidney is made up of 1.2 million functional units called nephrons. Most (80%) of cortical nephrons have short loops of Henle. The juxtamedullary nephrons (20%) have long loops of Henle which pass into the inner medulla, and are primarily concerned with the countercurrent exchange mechanism to establish a concentration gradient within the renal medulla. Renal blood flow accounts, for about 20% of cardiac output (625 ml/min to each kidney), this does not change with exercise and there is autoregulation over a range of blood pressures. The cortex receives the majority of the renal blood flow, in order to form an ultrafiltrate.

SCC pp 117–122

A **20.** **A.** false **B.** false **C.** false **D.** true **E.** true

Glomerular filtration rate (GFR) is measured using the Fick principle for the clearance of inulin. Inulin is a polysaccharide of MW 5500 Daltons which is injected into the body and filtered. It is not re-absorbed or secreted by the kidney, allowing measurement of urinary inulin to be used to calculate the filtration rate. Creatinine clearance is used to give an estimate of GFR, but since creatinine is secreted to a small degree by the tubules, it tends to over estimate the value for GFR. Renal plasma flow is calculated by the clearance of para-amino hippuric acid (PAH). Renal blood flow is large leading to small differences between arterial and venous blood in oxygen content. Oxygen consumption in the cortex is twenty times that in the medulla due to active transport in the tubules.

SCC pp 117–122

A **21.** **A.** false **B.** false **C.** false **D.** true **E.** true

Renin is released from the juxtaglomerula apparatus in the renal cortex. Renin is a proteolytic enzyme that is released into the plasma when the body sodium content decreases. Renin also exists in the brain, heart and adrenal gland. Its substrate is an α_2-globulin, angiotensinogen, liberating an decapeptide (angiotensin I) and an octapeptide (angiotensin II) via a converting enzyme. Angiotensin II acts on the zone glomerulose of the adrenal cortex to liberate aldosterone. This in turn acts on the kidney to increase salt and water retention. Angiotensin II has effects on the cardiovascular, renal and CNS (causing vasoconstriction) and is broken down in the liver.

SCC pp 117–122

A 22. **A.** true   **B.** false   **C.** false   **D.** true   **E.** false

Hypertension can cause a diuresis by increasing medullary blood flow and reducing the concentration gradient. Carbonic anhydrase inhibitors e.g. acetozolamide produce a weak diuresis with high pH, low ammonia and increased bicarbonate loop diuretics, such as frusemide the Na^+ Cl^- co-transport system in the thick ascending loop of Henle. Amiloride is not an aldosterone antagonist (spironolactone is an aldosterone antagonist).

SCC pp 203–205

Principles of Intensive Care

Answers

A 1. **A.** false **B.** false **C.** true **D.** false **E.** true

Silicone catheters are non-thrombogenic. 10–15% of central venous pressure (CVP) catheters become colonised. The insertion point for a subclavian line is at the junction between the medial 1/3 and the lateral 2/3 of the clavicle. The femoral vein lies within the sheath medial to the artery.

Surgery 2000 18: 2; 56A–C   **SCC** pp 211–217

A 2. **A.** true **B.** true **C.** true **D.** true **E.** false

Indications for intra-cranial pressure (ICP) monitoring are when clinical signs are obscured (drugs), to assess need for intervention (head injury, infection), intensive care unit (ICU) management of head injury and calculation of cerebral perfusion pressure (CPP)

$$CPP = \text{mean arterial pressure} - ICP$$

ICP measurement can be extradural, subdural, subarachnoid or via a lateral ventricle catheter.

Surgical Critical Care Ashford R, Evans N. GMM Ltd. London, 2001.

SCC pp 225–227

A 3. **A.** true **B.** false **C.** true **D.** false **E.** true

Tracheo-innominate artery erosion (TIAE) carries a mortality when treated urgently by ligation of the TIA of 75%. The anterior jugular vein is the vein most likely to cause bleeding problems.

Other complications:

- IMMED: haemorrhage, air embolus, local structure damage, apnoea, misplacement
- Continuing care: infection, tracheitis, tracheal stenosis & necrosis, tube blockage/displacement, surgical

emphysema, pneumothorax, decannulation problems and fistulae

Surgical Critical Care Ashford R, Evans N. GMM Ltd. London, 2001.

SCC pp 217–220

A 4. **A.** false **B.** true **C.** true **D.** true **E.** false

The cricothyroid membrane is superior to the cricoid cartilage, inferior to the thyroid cartilage. Emergency procedures have a complication rate five times that of elective.

SCC pp 220–221

A 5. **A.** true **B.** true **C.** true **D.** true **E.** true

All the above plus AV fistula, drugs being given in error through it, and compromise to distal flow as well as infection.

SCC pp 211–217

A 6. **A.** true **B.** false **C.** false **D.** false **E.** false

The internal jugular vein (IJV) is intimately associated with the carotid artery throughout its course, lying initially posterior to it and then antero-lateral within the carotid sheath. The IJV is superficial in the upper part of its course, covered by sternomastoid muscle in the middle third is again superficial in the lower third as it splits the sternal and clavicular heads of that muscle. Cannulation of the middle third requires the operator to traverse the sternomastoid muscle which can be unpleasant for the patient when awake. Arrhythmias occur because of guide wire stimulation of the right atrium and ventricle and is equally likely if the wire is advanced too far. Electrocardiogram (ECG) monitoring should always be available for this reason during central line insertion.

SCC pp 211–214

A 7. **A.** false **B.** false **C.** false **D.** false **E.** true

In patients with cerebral impairment and raised ICP, head neutral or head down tilt should be limited to the minimum possible for the procedure. However continuing with head up tilt risks the development of air embolus, particularly if the patient is dehydrated and should never be attempted. A low approach to the IJV reduces the chance of arterial puncture but increases the incidence of pneumothorax. The subclavian approach should not be attempted if the patient has a bleeding diathesis since it cannot be compressed in cases of vessel rupture. The external jugular vein (EJV) has valves which prohibit the passage of a guide wire. IJV on the right side is the site of choice but a catheter placed too far will risk intra-cardiac rupture.

SCC pp 211–214

Section 2 – Vivas

Q 1.   What clinical features may indicate poor peripheral perfusion?

Q 2.   What complications may arise following thoracic surgery?

Q 3.   What post-operative arrhythmias commonly occur following cardiac surgery and how would you manage them?

Q 4.   What are the causes of pulseless electrical activity (PEA)?

Q 5.   What are the causes of anaemia in the critically ill patient and when would you transfuse them?

Q 6.   What is Starling's Law of the heart?

Q 7.   What information can be obtained by pulmonary artery catheterisation in the critically ill patient?

Q 8.   What are the indications for pulmonary artery catheterisation in the critically ill patient?

Q 9.   What are the complications of blood transfusion?

Q 10. How would you manage the acute onset of atrial fibrillation (AF)?

Q 11. How would you treat acute pulmonary oedema?

Q 12. How would you manage the acutely unwell patient with sudden onset chest pain radiating to the back and an absent right brachial and radial pulse?

Q 13. Define disseminated intravascular coagulation (DIC). What are the causes and what haematological results would you expect in DIC?

Q 14. **What are the indications for an intra-aortic balloon pump (IABP)?**

Q 15. **What are the potential complications of central vein cannulation?**

Q 16. **How would you optimise cardiac output in the hypotensive patient?**

Q 1. How would you interpret a chest radiograph in a critically ill surgical patient?

Q 2. How would you diagnose adult respiratory distress syndrome (ARDS) in a ventilator dependent post-operative surgical patient?

Q 3. How is respiration controlled?

Q 4. What is involved in initiating a breath?

Q 5. How is respiration affected by a) exercise b) general anaesthesia c) hypovolaemia d) altitude?

Q 6. What is functional residual capacity (FRC) and why is it important?

Q 7. What is measured using a spirometer?

Q 8. What dynamic tests of respiratory function do you know?

Q 9. What is meant by respiratory compliance?

Q 10. How do ventilation and perfusion vary with spontaneous and mechanical ventilation? What do you understand by the terms 'shunt' and 'dead space'?

Q 11. How would you go about interpreting arterial blood gas (ABG) analysis?

Q 12. How would you classify hypoxia?

Q 13. Which patients are at risk of post-operative hypoxaemia? What methods are available to deliver oxygen to a spontaneously breathing patient after surgery?

Q 14. How would you classify respiratory failure, and what are the signs?

Q 15. What are the indications for intubation and mechanical ventilation?

Q 16. What are the effects of mechanical ventilation?

Q 17. What modes of mechanical ventilation do you know? Which of these modes are used for weaning?

Q 18. Why is it important to maintain adequate lung volume? What methods do you know for optimising lung volume?

Q 19. What factors affect the ability to wean from mechanical ventilation?

Q 20. What are the causes of airway obstruction? How may these be managed?

Q 21. What are the principle causes of ARDS? What clinical findings make up the diagnosis?

Q 22. Describe the pathophysiological processes responsible for ARDS? What is the prognosis?

Q 23. What are the objectives for respiratory support in a patient with ARDS? What mechanisms are there to maintain adequate oxygenation?

Q 1. What are the indications for a computed tomography (CT) scan following a head injury?

Q 2. What type of injuries are possible to blood vessels and what are their sequelae?

Q 3. What are the causes of raised intracranial pressure (ICP) after head injury?

Q 4. What are the indications for urgent surgical exploration in thoracic trauma?

Q 5. How do you decide how much fluid to give a patient with major burns?

Q 6. How do you diagnose and treat fat embolism syndrome (FES)?

Q 7. What features of burn injuries would make you suspect an inhalational injury and how would you manage it?

Q 8. How would you assess the severity of a head injury?

Q 9. What are the causes of massive haemoptysis and how would you manage a patient with it?

Q 10. How would you manage a patient with acute hepatic failure (AHF)?

Q 11. What are the clinical features of a raised ICP?

Q 12. How would you manage a patient with a spinal cord injury?

Q 13. What methods are employed to try to prevent multi-organ dysfunction syndrome (MODS)?

Q 14. How would you manage a patient with a severe upper gastrointestinal bleed?

Q 15. How would you manage a patient with blunt chest trauma?

Q 16. **What is systemic inflammatory response syndrome (SIRS) and how would you diagnose it?**

Q 17. **What is MODS?**

Q 18. **What are the principles of management in MODS?**

Q 19. **What are the advantages and disadvantages of enteral nutrition?**

Q 20. **What are the advantages and disadvantages of parenteral nutrition?**

Q 21. **How may nutrition regimens be tailored to patients with organ dysfunction?**

Q 22. **What are the daily nutritional requirements of patients and how may these vary with critical illness?**

Q 1. What are the differences between sepsis, severe sepsis and septic shock?

Q 2. What are the features of occult intra-abdominal sepsis and how would you diagnose and treat it?

Q 1. What are the principles for the safe transfer of the critically ill surgical patient?

Q 2. What are the basics of successful clinical monitoring of the critically ill patient?

Q 3. What parameters would make you consider early referral to critical care?

Q 4. What are the principles of analgesia in the multiple injured patient?

Q 5. What reasons might you want a surgical patient to go to intensive therapy unit (ITU) electively?

Q 6. What is meant by scoring systems for intensive care unit (ICU) patients? What scoring systems do you know?

Q 1. What are the complications of inserting an intercostal chest drain?

Q 2. What are the indications for tracheostomy and what are its advantages?

Q 3. Describe how you would perform a venous cut-down of the long saphenous vein at the ankle.

Q 4. What are the findings for a diagnostic peritoneal lavage (DPL) to be positive?

Q 5. Why might you consider monitoring intra-abdominal pressure (IAP)?

Q 6. What is a chest drain and how does it function?

Q 7. What are the indications and potential complications of central venous cannulation?

Q 8. Outline the relevant anatomy of a) the internal jugular vein (IJV) and b) the subclavian vein. Describe the technique used to cannulate each of these central veins.

Q 1. **What clinical features may indicate poor peripheral perfusion?**

A 1. Classically poor peripheral perfusion is indicated by cool clammy skin with poor capillary filling and collapsed veins. Other indicators are confusion, decreased peripheral temperature, oliguria or anuria, metabolic acidosis, a low volume pulse and peripheral cyanosis.

SCC pp 15–20

Q 2. **What complications may arise following thoracic surgery?**

A 2. **Intrathoracic bleeding**
Usually occurs from lung parenchyma or bronchial vessels and may present with clinical features of hypovolaemia. It is usually detectable from drains. Re-operation is required if there is rapid blood loss via chest drain, a significant intrapleural collection on chest X-ray, persisting hypovolaemia despite transfusion or hypoxia due to compression of the underlying lung.

Sputum retention and atelectasis
Presents as tachypnoea and hypoxia. Examination usually shows reduced bilateral basal air entry. Prevention is preferred to treatment. The mainstay of treatment is chest physiotherapy, but tracheostomy and suction may be required. Antibiotics are reserved for those with proven pneumonia.

Air leak
These presents as a persist air leak or bubbling of chest drain and usually settle spontaneously over 2–3 days. They may require suction on pleural drains. Apposition of lung to parietal pleura encourages efficient healing.

Bronchopleural fistula
Fistulae are seen in 2% of patients undergoing pneumonectomy. They usually occur as a result form a leak from a suture line, and

occurs particularly in those with factors impairing wound healing. They most commonly occur 7–10 days after surgery presenting with sudden breathlessness and expectoration of bloodstained fluid. Treatment is to lie the patient with operated side downwards, oxygen and chest drain, thoracotomy and repair of fistula may also be required.

SCC pp 49–55

Q 3. **What post-operative arrhythmias commonly occur following cardiac surgery and how would you manage them?**

A 3. Atrial tachyarrhythmias occur with an incidence of between 17 and 33%, and generally occur between days 2 and 3. Atrial fibrillation (AF) is the most common, is usually symptomatic but often self-limiting. It may cause haemodynamic compromise or thromboembolic events. The treatment depends on haemodynamics. For the haemodynamically stable a β-blocker is indicated, for the haemodynamically unstable, DC cardioversion is employed first then rate control drugs (metoprolol, digoxin, verapamil).

Sustained ventricular tachyarrhythmias are uncommon after surgery (0.4–1.4%). These arrhythmias are associated with haemodynamic instability, electrolyte disturbances, hypoxia and graft occlusion. These are associated with poorer short and long term prognosis with a hospital mortality of upto 50%. Acute treatment may require lidocaine or amiodarone. Ventricular tachycardia may progress to ventricular fibrillation requiring defibrillation. Isolated premature ventricular complexes are not uncommon, often associated with electrolyte imbalance and do not require acute treatment.

SCC p 51

Q 4. **What are the causes of pulseless electrical activity (PEA)?**

A 4. Pulseless electrical activity (PEA) was known as electromechanical dissociation (EMD). It is the presence of an electrical cardiac rhythm in the absence of a cardiac output. Causes are divided into primary and secondary (*Table 1.1*)

Table 1.1 Primary and secondary causes of PEA

Primary PEA	Secondary PEA
Myocardial infarction	Tension pneumothorax
Drugs	Hypovolaemic shock
■ β-blockers	Cardiac tamponade
■ Calcium antagonists	Pulmonary embolus
Electrolyte imbalance	Cardiac rupture
■ Hyperkalaemia	
■ Hypocalcaemia	

SCC pp 11–15

Q 5. **What are the causes of anaemia in the critically ill patient and when would you transfuse them?**

A 5. Anaemia can be due to bleeding (occult or overt), anaemia of critical illness, or in the very young due to repeated blood sampling. Occult bleeding can be into the skull, thorax, abdomen, retroperitoneal space, pelvis, limbs for closed long bone fractures or at the scene of an accident. Anaemia of critical illness is due to bone marrow suppression, decreased erythropoetin production or an impaired bone marrow response to erythropoetin.

Transfusion is necessary when there is evidence of impaired perfusion. There is no single transfusion trigger figure but the following give an idea when transfusion is necessary: haemoglobin, haematocrit, ongoing haemorrhage, symptomatic anaemia, perfusion impairments and impaired oxygenation. A lower threshold for transfusion is necessary with extremes of age.

SCC pp 36–41

Q 6. **What is Starling's Law of the heart?**

A 6. Starling's Law describes the relationship between preload or filling pressure and stroke volume. The force of myocardial muscle contraction is proportional to the amount of stretch in the cardiac muscle fibres prior to contraction. Thus, in the normal heart stroke, volume increases as the end-diastolic volume increases (*Fig. 1.1*). The ventricular function curve is displaced upwards (increased contractility) by sympathetic activation including positive inotropes (e.g. dobutamine, adrenaline) and displaced downwards (decreased contractility) by hypoxia,

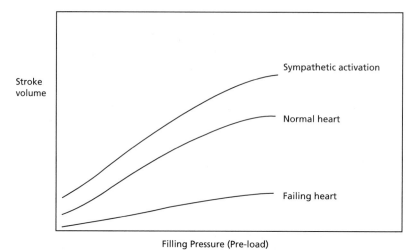

Fig. 1.1 Ventricular function curves demonstrating the relationship between stroke volume and preload in the normal, failing and stimulated heart.

acidosis and negatively inotropic drugs (e.g. β-blockers and calcium antagonists).

The relationship between preload and stroke volume persists in the failing heart. Indeed, it acts as one of the compensatory mechanisms in heart failure that initially maintains stroke volume. A reduced stroke volume results in an increased amount of blood in the ventricle at end-diastole. The amount of stretch within the ventricular muscle fibres is therefore increased and through Starling's Law, myocardial contractility is increased, restoring stroke volume.

In the failing heart, however, the left ventricular function curve is flattened (*Fig. 1.1*) such that increasing left atrial filling pressure, the preload of the left ventricle, (above about 20 mmHg) does not produce a further increase in stroke volume, but does predispose to the development of pulmonary venous hypertension and pulmonary oedema.

SCC pp 3–4

Q 7. **What information can be obtained by pulmonary artery catheterisation in the critically ill patient?**

A 7. During catheterisation of the right heart and pulmonary artery, pressures are transduced directly from the catheter tip through the fluid-filled lumen: central venous pressure (CVP), right ventricular pressure, pulmonary artery pressure, pulmonary artery occlusion pressure (PAOP). Blood can be aspirated from the distal port or the right atrial port of the catheter to measure blood oxygen saturations from the right heart and pulmonary artery. Cardiac output and systemic vascular resistance (SVR) can be estimated indirectly from information gained during right heart catheterisation.

The CVP and the PAOP provide an objective measure of the filling pressure or preload of the right and left ventricles, respectively. Right ventricular and pulmonary artery pressure indicate whether or not pulmonary hypertension is present. A 'step-up' in blood oxygen saturations between the right atrium and right ventricle indicates that oxygenated blood is entering the right ventricle (a left to right shunt) and is consistent with a ventricular septal defect (VSD), which may occur acutely after myocardial infarction.

Cardiac output is estimated by thermodilution. A known volume (typically 10 ml) of cold crystalloid is injected into the right atrial port of the pulmonary artery catheter. A thermistor at the catheter tip measures the resultant transient temperature decrease in the pulmonary artery. The area under the curve when fall in temperature is plotted against time correlates with cardiac output, which is calculated by computer.

SVR can be calculated from aortic pressure, right atrial pressure and cardiac output.

$$SVR = \frac{80\ (\text{mean aortic pressure} - \text{mean right atrial pressure})}{\text{cardiac output}}$$

SCC pp 18–20

Q 8. **What are the indications for pulmonary artery catheterisation in the critically ill patient?**

A 8. The indications for pulmonary artery catheterisation can be broadly divided into scenarios requiring measurement of the PAOP, cardiac output and SVR, and blood oxygen saturations (*see* Question 2 in this section and *Table 1.2*).

Table 1.2 Indications for pulmonary artery catheterisation

Measurement of PAOP to determine volume status and optimise cardiac output:
- Oliguria
- Hypotension
- RV infarction
- Cardiogenic shock
- Septic shock
- Adult respiratory distress syndrome (ARDS)

Measurement of cardiac output/SVR to guide inotropic therapy:
- Cardiogenic shock
- Septic shock

Measurement of right heart blood O_2 saturations:
- Diagnosis of left to right shunt (VSD)
- Mixed venous (PA) O_2 concentration needed for some measures of cardiac output

PAOP

The accurate assessment of volume status is central to the appropriate management of the critically ill patient. Measurement of the PAOP is therefore indicated when volume status remains uncertain after clinical evaluation. Clinical assessment of volume status may be particularly difficult in the presence of chronic lung disease and tricuspid regurgitation. Furthermore, if there is a disparity between the function of the right and left ventricle (right ventricular infarction, pulmonary embolism, cor pulmonale, left ventricular disease), the filling pressure of the right heart (CVP) may not reflect the filling pressure of the left heart. In these circumstances, the CVP will not be an accurate guide to volume status and measurement of the PAOP is indicated.

A normal PAOP is about 8–12 mmHg. A low value implies hypovolaemia. Pulmonary oedema in the presence of a low PAOP indicates ARDS. An elevated PAOP implies volume overload.

In addition to its diagnostic purpose, PAOP can also be used to guide fluid administration in patients who are at risk of developing volume overload such as the elderly or those with a history of heart disease.

Cardiac output

Measurement of cardiac output is useful both as a diagnostic aid and to monitor therapy in the critically ill patient. A low cardiac output in the hypotensive patient is consistent with cardiogenic shock and indicates the need for inotropic support, while a high cardiac output is consistent with septic shock.

SVR

In the clinical setting, the determination of SVR is often used together with cardiac output and PAOP to assist in the diagnosis of the shocked patient (*Table 1.3*). A low SVR is characteristic of septic shock, while the SVR is usually raised in cardiogenic shock and hypovolaemia.

Serial measurements of PAOP, cardiac output and SVR can be used to monitor the effects of fluid administration and inotropic therapy.

Blood oxygen saturations

The differential diagnosis of the patient in cardiogenic shock after acute myocardial infarction includes VSD and mitral regurgitation due to papillary muscle rupture. Differentiating between the two may be difficult because both cause similar clinical presentations and a pansystolic murmur. If the diagnosis cannot be made by echo, then blood oxygen saturations can be measured from the right ventricle and right atrium. A 'step-up' in oxygen saturation in the right ventricle (oxygen saturation higher than the right atrium) would be consistent with a VSD.

Mixed venous (pulmonary artery) blood oxygen saturation measurement is required for estimation of cardiac output by the Fick method.

Table 1.3 The differential diagnosis of shock using haemodynamic parameters obtained from Swan-Ganz catheterisation

	PAOP	*Cardiac index*	*SVR*
Hypovolaemia	↓	↓	↑
Cardiogenic shock	↑	↓	↑
Septic shock	↓	↑	↓

PAOP = pulmonary artery occlusion pressure; SVR = systemic vascular resistance; Normal values: PCWP 8–12 mmHg; Cardiac index 2.5–4.0 l/min/m^2; SVR 770–1500 dynes s/cm^5

SCC pp 18–20

A 9. The possible complications of blood transfusion are: precipitation of heart failure, febrile reaction, haemolytic transfusion reaction, transmission of infection, hyperkalaemia, hypocalcaemia, thrombocytopenia, disseminated intravascular coagulation (DIC), hypothermia.

Haemolytic transfusion reactions are usually due to ABO incompatibility caused by administrative error. They should be managed by stopping the blood transfusion, checking patient identity against the blood unit, returning the blood unit to the haematology laboratory with a sample of clotted blood and ethylene diamintetraacetic acid (EDTA) sample. Severe reactions may require the administration of fluid, adrenaline, antihistamine and steroids as for anaphylactic shock. Milder febrile reactions are usually due to antibodies against white cells.

A number of infections (viruses, bacteria, protozoa) can be transmitted by blood transfusions. Most concern surrounds the transmission of viral infections including hepatitis B & C, human immunodeficiency virus (HIV), Epstein-Barr virus (EBV), and cytomegalo virus (CMV). Antibodies against hepatitis B & C, and HIV are screened for in blood donated in the UK.

Massive transfusion (defined as a transfusion volume equal to the patient's own blood volume within 24 hours) may be associated with several complications. Stored blood contains few platelets and reduced concentrations of factors V and VIII. 'Dilutional' thrombocytopenia and clotting factor deficiency may therefore occur during massive transfusion. The platelet count, INR and activated partial thromboplastin time (APTT) should be monitored, and the administration of platelets and fresh frozen plasma may be required. The plasma potassium concentration increases during storage as potassium leaks out of the red cells. Plasma calcium levels may be reduced by binding of ionised calcium by citrate added to stored blood. Hypocalcaemia and hyperkalaemia may therefore occasionally result after massive transfusion. Hypothermia may result from the rapid transfusion of blood and blood warmers should be used during rapid massive transfusion.

SCC pp 38–41

Q 10. How would you manage the acute onset of atrial fibrillation (AF)?

A 10. AF is characterised by the absence of a P wave before each QRS complex and irregularity of the ventricular (QRS) response (*Fig. 1.2*).

Management includes the identification and correction of reversible causes such as electrolyte imbalance. Further management depends upon whether haemodynamic compromise is present and on the ventricular rate. If significant haemodynamic compromise is thought to be caused by the new occurrence of AF, then DC cardioversion should be performed urgently.

If the patient is not significantly compromised, then he can either be managed with ventricular rate control or by elective cardioversion. Digoxin, β-blockers and verapamil can be used for rate control. Cardioversion may be attempted chemically or electrically. A number of anti-arrhythmic drugs can be used to cardiovert AF to sinus rhythm, but success is limited and they all carry the risk of pro-arrhythmia, particularly if the heart is not structurally normal. Amiodarone and β-blockers are the safest drugs in the structurally abnormal heart. DC cardioversion carries a higher success rate. Cardioversion can be performed without anticoagulation if the onset of AF occurred within 48 hours, as

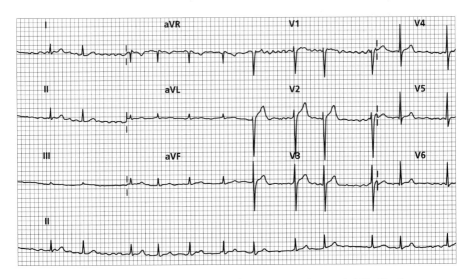

Fig. 1.2 Electrocardiogram (ECG) demonstrating atrial fibrillation.

the risk of left atrial thrombus formation is low within this time frame. Thereafter, 4 weeks of warfarin prior to cardioversion (as an outpatient) is recommended. All patients with persistent AF, except those aged <65 years with lone AF, should be considered for warfarin to prevent stroke.

SCC pp 20–21

Q 11. How would you treat acute pulmonary oedema?

A 11. Reassure the patient. Sit him up. Monitor ECG and oxygen saturations. Administer high flow oxygen via a rebreathing bag. Give intravenous opiate (e.g. diamorphine 2.5–5 mg) and anti-emetic (e.g. metaclopramide 10 mg). Opiates act as venodilators, reducing preload, and also as an anxiolytic. Administer intravenous diuretic (e.g. frusemide 40 mg). Acutely, this acts as a venodilator prior to the onset of its diuretic effect. If the patient is not hypotensive, initiate an intravenous nitrate infusion. Again, this causes vasodilatation and reduces preload. As pulmonary venous pressure falls to the threshold at which plasma oncotic pressure favours resorption of fluid, pulmonary oedema begins to resolve. If the patient is hypotensive (cardiogenic shock), inotropes (e.g. dobutamine 2.5–15 μg/kg/min) should be initiated. The dose is tailored to achieve a blood pressure capable of perfusing the major organs. Clinically, this is reflected by a satisfactory urine output.

SCC pp 33–35

Q 12. How would you manage the acutely unwell patient with sudden onset chest pain radiating to the back and an absent right brachial and radial pulse?

A 12. The likely diagnosis is aortic dissection, but myocardial ischaemia with right subclavian artery stenosis due to atherosclerosis, and emboli to the brachial artery and a coronary artery due to left atrial thrombus or endocarditis, are possible. Monitoring of vital signs, ECG and oxygen saturations should be performed. Oxygen and opiate analgesia should be administered. Examination of the patient should focus on determining the contralateral BP, the presence or absence of the other peripheral pulses and of aortic regurgitation.

Blood tests will include full blood count (FBC), U & E, and cross-match. Initial investigations may provide supportive evidence for the diagnosis of aortic dissection. A 12-lead ECG should be performed. However, any of these scenarios may produce ST segment changes of ischaemia or infarction. In aortic dissection, this is caused if a coronary artery ostium is disrupted by the dissection flap. Transthoracic echo may demonstrate the dissection flap, and will also demonstrate the presence of aortic regurgitation and pericardial effusion, both consistent with aortic dissection. CXR may reveal a widened mediastinum and/or a pericardial effusion in cases of aortic dissection.

The definitive diagnosis is usually made by either contrast-enhanced CT scan, magnetic resonance imaging (MRI) or transoesophageal echo (TOE). This depends largely on local availability and expertise. CT scanning is readily available and non-invasive. MRI tends to be less readily available and it presents difficulties in monitoring of the acutely ill patient. TOE requires an experienced operator, but can be performed on the ward or in the anaesthetic room and provides additional information about the presence of aortic regurgitation, pericardial effusion, left ventricular function and relationship of the coronary ostea to the dissection flap. Aortography is now rarely used because it is invasive and potentially complicated by catheters entering the false lumen.

Further management is dependent upon the site of the dissection. Stanford type A dissections involve the ascending aorta and are managed surgically, while type B dissections do not involve the ascending aorta and are managed medically unless complications ensue. The mainstay of medical management is control of blood pressure using agents such as intravenous labetalol and sodium nitroprusside to obtain acute control of BP (target 100–120 mmHg systolic), with the addition of oral agents (e.g. β-blockers, calcium blockers, ACE inhibitors) thereafter. If distal dissection is complicated by rupture, aneurysm formation, vital organ or limb ischaemia, continued pain, or retrograde progression into the ascending aorta, then surgery is indicated.

SCC pp 26–27

Q 13. Define disseminated intravascular coagulation (DIC). What are the causes and what haematological results would you expect in DIC?

A 13. DIC is characterised by activation of the clotting cascades with generation of fibrin, consumption of clotting factors and platelets, and secondary activation of fibrinolysis leading to production of fibrinogen degradation products (FDPs). Clinically, it may be asymptomatic manifest only on blood investigations, or may cause bleeding, or tissue ischaemia due to vessel occlusion by fibrin and platelets.

DIC may be caused by Gram-negative, meningococcal and staphylococcal septicaemia, tissue damage after trauma, burns or surgery, malignancy, haemolytic blood transfusion reactions, falciparum malaria, snake bites, and obstetric conditions such as placental abruption and amniotic fluid embolism.

The prothrombin time (or INR), APTT, and thrombin time are prolonged. The fibrinogen level and platelet count are low. High levels of FDPs are present. There may be fragmented red cells on the blood film due to red cell damage during passage through fibrin webs in the circulation.

SCC pp 47–49

Q 14. What are the indications for an intra-aortic balloon pump (IABP)?

A 14. The intra-aortic ballon pump (IABP) augments diastolic pressure and reduces afterload resulting in increased coronary and cerebral perfusion and a reduction in myocardial oxygen demand. The main indication for an IABP is supportive therapy prior to a definitive procedure. Most commonly, this is in the haemodynamically compromised patient with a post-myocardial infarct VSD or mitral regurgitation due to papillary muscle rupture, or in a patient with ongoing myocardial ischaemia despite maximal medical therapy as a bridge to coronary angioplasty or coronary artery bypass graft surgery. IABP may also be used post-operatively, usually after cardiac surgery, in patients with left ventricular dysfunction. IABP may also be placed prophylactically in high-risk coronary angioplasty. IABP is contra-indicated in patients with significant aortic regurgitation (which it exacerbates), aortic dissection, aortic aneurysm, and severe peripheral vascular disease.

SCC p 8

Q 15. What are the potential complications of central vein cannulation?

A 15. These are:

- arterial puncture, which may result in haemothorax
- pneumothorax
- infection (localised or systemic)
- endocarditis (with chronic central venous cannulation)
- neurological injury
- air embolism.

SCC pp 211–214

Q 16. How would you optimise cardiac output in the hypotensive patient?

A 16. The specific management of the hypotensive patient is clearly partly dependent upon the cause of the haemodynamic compromise. For example, if the hypotension is secondary to haemorrhage, then volume replacement with blood is the treatment. The commonest cause of cardiogenic shock is acute myocardial infarction, which is managed with aspirin, coronary reperfusion by thrombolysis or angioplasty, and inotropes. In the critically ill patient, hypotension may be multifactorial with hypovolaemia, sepsis and left ventricular dysfunction contributing. Certain principles of supportive management can be outlined.

Assess and optimise volume status
Clinical assessment of volume status comprises searching for a history of blood or volume loss, examining the patient for signs of hypovolaemia or volume overload, examining fluid balance charts, and reviewing a CXR (*Table 1.4*).

Table 1.4 Clinical assessment of volume status in the hypotensive or oliguric patient

	Hypovolaemia	*Volume overload*
History	Poor intake or volume loss, e.g. GI bleed, vomiting	Known heart failure or suggestive history
Examination	Postural hypotension, jugular venous pressure (JVP)↓, clear lungs, no oedema	JVP↑, S3, crepitations, oedema
Fluid balance	Negative	Positive
CXR	No pulmonary oedema	Pulmonary oedema

S3 = third heart sound.

Invasive monitoring

If volume status remains uncertain after clinical assessment, CVP and/or Swan-Ganz catheter insertion is indicated. In most circumstances, a right-sided filling pressure (CVP) of 10–12 mmHg and a left-sided filling pressure (PAOP) of 16–18 mmHg indicates an appropriate preload to optimise cardiac output. If the filling pressure is too low, fluid should be administered until the PAOP is optimised.

Assess the need for inotropes

Inotropes are indicated if hypotension is present in the presence of a high PAOP (i.e. the patient is volume overloaded or in cardiogenic shock), or if hypotension persists after correction of hypovolaemia. Assessment of cardiac output and SVR may assist in the diagnosis of the cause of shock (*Table 1.3*) and in the choice of the appropriate inotropes.

In *cardiogenic shock*, the cardiac output is low and SVR high. In theory therefore the ideal inotrope in these circumstances would increase cardiac output while decreasing SVR. Dobutamine has these properties, at least at lower doses. At higher doses, vasoconstriction and an increase in SVR can occur.

In *septic shock*, cardiac output is usually high and SVR low. Vasoconstricting inotropes e.g. adrenaline or noradrenaline are appropriate.

Assess the need for IABP

IABP insertion is particularly indicated as supportive therapy prior to a definitive procedure e.g. in a patient with a post-myocardial infarct VSD or mitral regurgitation due to papillary muscle rupture.

Treat associated arrhythmias

Arrhythmias, particularly AF, are common in the critically ill patient. If the main cause of haemodynamic compromise is thought to be the new occurrence of AF, then DC cardioversion should be performed urgently. Agents such as amiodarone can be used in an attempt to maintain sinus rhythm. More commonly, AF is one of a number of contributing factors and can be managed by control of the ventricular response rate with drugs such as digoxin.

Table 1.5 Summary of the optimisation of cardiac output in the critically ill patient

Optimise preload	If hypovolaemic, replace fluids
	If volume overloaded, IV glyceryl trinitrate (GTN) and IV furosemide
Optimise afterload	Sodium nitroprusside or hydralazine
Indications for inotropes	If remains hypotensive despite adequate filling pressures:
	Dobutamine ± dopamine for cardiogenic shock
	Noradrenaline/adrenaline for septic shock
Indications for IABP	Acute mitral regurgitation or VSD
Treat AF	Control ventricular response rate
	Preserved LV function: β-blockers, verapamil, diltiazem
	Impaired LV function: digoxin, amiodarone

SCC pp 15–20

Answers

Q 1. **How would you interpret a chest radiograph in a critically ill surgical patient?**

A 1. A system is necessary to ensure that all the appropriate parts of a chest X-ray are reviewed and nothing is missed.

- Is this the correct patient?
- Are there any potentially life threatening abnormalities (e.g. large pneumothorax)
- Assess external lines and leads
  - Central line
  - Endotracheal tube (ETT)
  - Electrocardiogram (ECG)
  - Chest drains
  - Pacemaker
- Assess technical aspects
  - Left and right correctly labelled
  - Centering of the film
  - Lung volumes
  - Penetration
- The lungs
  - Pulmonary vascular pattern
  - Hila
  - Costophrenic region
- The mediastinum
  - Trachea central or deviated
  - Left and right heart borders
  - Heart size
- The soft tissue and bones
  - Fractures
  - Free air under the diaphragm

SCC pp 75–76

Q 2. **How would you diagnose adult respiratory distress syndrome (ARDS) in a ventilator dependent post-operative surgical patient?**

A 2. Adult respiratory distress syndrome (ARDS) is partly determined by the underlying or precipitating condition. The pathology is an increase in permeability of the alveolar capillary membrane. The diagnostic criteria for ARDS are given in the *Table 2.1*.

Table 2.1 Diagnostic criteria for ARDS

Acute onset
Oxygenation $PaO_2/F_iO_2 \leq 200$
CXR – bilateral infiltrates
Pulmonary artery occlusion pressure (PAOP) < 18 mmHg
No clinical evidence of increasing left atrial pressure

SCC pp 91–96

Q 3. **How is respiration controlled?**

A 3. Respiration is under the control of the central nervous system (CNS), voluntary control by the cortex and automatic control by the medulla. Inspiratory and expiratory neurones in the reticular formation of the medulla provide the 'pacemaker' for the respiratory cycle. The aim of respiration is to adjust ventilation to maintain appropriate levels of PaO_2, $PaCO_2$ and pH. There are several mechanisms providing the CNS with feedback about these respiratory parameters:

1. The central chemoreceptors lie close to the floor of the fourth ventricle and are intimately associated with the respiratory centre.
   - These receptors are sensitive to changes in the pH of the interstitial fluid that surrounds them
   - Hydrogen (H^+) and bicarbonate (HCO_3^-) diffuse slowly between blood and the cerebrospinal fluid (CSF), but carbon dioxide (CO_2) moves freely, allowing rapid reflection of blood CO_2 in the CSF
   - ↑ CO_2 translates to an exaggerated ↓ pH (since the CSF has little buffering capacity)
   - The pH change is detected by the central chemoreceptors and stimulates the respiratory centre to increase minute volume

- The CO_2 change in CSF is eventually buffered by the slower diffusion of HCO_3^- across the blood brain barrier
2. The peripheral chemoreceptors in the aorta and carotid bodies are sensitive to the PaO_2 of arterial blood and start discharging once the PaO_2 falls below 13 kPa (in healthy adults), causing an increase in the minute ventilation.

CO_2 homeostasis is usually the predominant influence on the control of ventilation. The role of O_2 becomes important during acute hypoxia e.g. chest infection or patients with CO_2 retention e.g. chronic bronchitis, who may rely on hypoxic drive (this, however represents only the minority of patients with COPD). The effects of hypercarbia and hypoxia summate in increasing minute volume.

The cerebral cortex is able to exert voluntary control over brainstem automatic ventilation. This can be modified by:

- Speech, eating, drinking and sleeping
- Sneezing, yawning and vomiting
- Activity and anticipation of exercise
- Fever and hypothermia

There are other feedback mechanisms to the CNS which influence respiration:

- Mechanoreceptors – these occur throughout the lungs and upper airway. The pulmonary stretch receptors protect against overdistention of the lung in the Hering-Breuer reflex. Impulses are carried in the vagus nerve to the CNS when lung volume reaches a critical level, preventing further inspiratory effort.
- Proprioceptors – these co-ordinate muscular activity and ventilation
- Temperature receptors – are responsible for the increase in respiratory rate with fever

SCC pp 60–61

Q 4. What is involved in initiating a breath?

A 4. Inspiration is an active process, initiated by inspiratory neurones in the respiratory centre, located in the floor of the fourth ventricle in the brainstem. To initiate a breath the respiratory centre stimulates the respiratory muscles via the cranial and spinal nerves.

1. The diaphragm is the principle muscle of respiration, accounting for about three quarters of the volume change.
    ■ As it contracts, it flattens, displacing the abdominal contents forward and downward. It can move up to 7 cm on deep inspiration.
    ■ ↑ Intra-thoracic volume leads to a ↓ intra-thoracic pressure (sub-atmospheric)
    ■ The transpulmonary pressure difference between atmospheric at the lips and the negative pressure in the alveoli drives the air into the lungs during inspiration
2. The accessory muscles of respiration are responsible for preventing the collapse of the airways caused by the negative intra-thoracic pressure during inspiration.
    ■ The external intercostal muscles contract to stabilise the chest wall, and contribute to the 'bucket handle' outer expansion of the lower ribs, which further increases intra-thoracic volume
    ■ The dilator muscles of the upper airway contract, maintaining patency during inspiration

The lungs and chest wall contain stretch and mechanoreceptors, which signal the inspiratory centre via the vagus nerve to end inspiration. The stretch receptors are also responsible for the Hering-Breuer reflex, which inhibits further inspiration when the lung is already inflated.

Expiration is usually a passive process of elastic recoil.

■ This is facilitated by the stored energy of the expanded chest wall following inspiration
■ Inspiratory neurones in the brainstem then start firing in response to afferent input from the stretch receptors on expiration

Expiration can also be active e.g. forced expiration during a cough, or increased airway resistance. Contraction of the abdominal muscles increases intra-abdominal pressure thrusting the diaphragm into the thoracic cavity. This process is enhanced by contraction of the internal intercostal muscles, reducing the capacity of the thoracic cavity.

Air is moved by convection from the lips to the terminal bronchioles and then by diffusion across the alveoli into the capillary network.

SCC p 59

Q 5. **How is respiration affected by a) exercise b) general anaesthesia c) hypovolaemia d) altitude?**

A 5. **Exercise**

Exercise stimulates reflex mechanisms which enhance cardio-respiratory performance. Anticipation of physical activity by the cortex stimulated increases respiratory centre activity. Pulmonary ventilation rises from a resting value of 6–8 l/min to values of upto 100 l/min in trained individuals. This increase in capacity is mediated by an increase in both respiratory frequency and tidal volume. Peripheral chemoreceptors play little role during this process as arterial pH, $PaCO_2$ and PaO_2 remain normal. Cardiac output also increases upto 30 l/min. Oxygen extraction increases secondary to metabolic acidosis produced by lactic acid formation from anaerobic metabolism in the tissues (mainly muscles). The accompanying temperature rise shifts the oxygen dissociation curve to the right. These measures combine to increase the tissue oxygen consumption from 300 ml/min at rest to up to 5 l/min during extreme exercise.

General anaesthesia

General anaesthesia produces a dose-dependent depression of respiration. The overall minute volume is reduced, mainly by a decreased tidal volume but with compensatory increase in respiratory rate. The respiratory pattern becomes almost exclusively diaphragmatic with little contribution from the accessory muscles of respiration. This results in elevated CO_2 levels in spontaneously breathing individuals. There is also a tendency towards hypoxaemia since functional residual capacity (FRC) and hypoxic pulmonary vasoconstriction (HPV) are both reduced. The chemoreceptor feedback to hypoxia and hypercarbia is depressed, further reducing ability of the CNS to respond to these changes.

Hypovolaemia

Loss of blood volume leads to tissue hypoxaemia due to hypoperfusion. The resultant metabolic acidosis secondary to circulatory failure produces a compensatory respiratory alkalosis by increasing the depth and rate of respiration. Peripheral chemoreceptors in the carotid body are directly stimulated by severe hypotension (systolic BP < 60 mmHg). Hypotension contributes to increased mismatch of ventilation : perfusion ratios and shunt formation, this exacerbates any existing hypoxaemia and further stimulates the respiratory centre by positive feedback.

Altitude

High altitude decreases barometric pressure, which in turn reduces the inspired oxygen partial pressure. This is a form of hypoxic hypoxaemia, and has a similar effect to breathing oxygen of low (<21%) concentration. The physiological changes that take place in order to adapt to these conditions is termed acclimatisation. Arterial hypoxaemia is detected by the peripheral chemoreceptors, which stimulate the respiratory centre. Alveolar ventilation can increase fivefold to levels above 20 l/min, reducing the $PaCO_2$ level by upto 80%. People living at high altitude have other 'adapted' physiological changes:

- Polycythaemia
- ↑ levels of 2,3-diphosphoglycerate (2,3-DPG) (causes right shift of ODC)
- Increased HPV (↑ pulmonary artery pressures)
- Increased mitochondrial density
- Increased maximum ventilatory capacity

SCC pp 60–65

Q 6. **What is functional residual capacity (FRC) and why is it important?**

A 6. FRC = 2.2 l: the volume of air remaining in the lung after tidal (V_t) expiration. This volume of air continues to take part in gaseous exchange at the end of expiration and allows a method for continuous oxygenation throughout the respiratory cycle. Its importance therefore is as an oxygen reserve, particularly when ventilation has stopped or is inefficient. A capacity is made up of two or more volumes. FRC is made up of residual volume (RV = 1.2 l) and expiratory reserve volume (ERV = 1 l). RV is the volume of air remaining in the lung after a maximal expiration, and is the minimum amount of air that can be left in the lung. ERV is the maximal volume of air that can be expelled after tidal (V_t) expiration.

Closing capacity (CC): this is the lung volume where small airways begin to collapse on expiration. Normally CC is greater than FRC.

However, if CC is less than FRC then there will be airway closure, leading to collapse during tidal (quiet) ventilation, resulting in arterial hypoxaemia. Thus, any factor that decreases FRC will increase the risk of airway closure and collapse (*Table 2.2*).

Table 2.2 Factors affecting FRC

Factors increasing FRC	*Factors decreasing FRC*
PEEP/CPAP	Extremes of age (very young and old)
Obstructive airways disease e.g. asthma, emphysema	Supine posture Anaesthesia Obesity Abdominal/Thoracic surgery* Pulmonary disease e.g. oedema or fibrosis

*The effects of surgery on lung volume can last for up to 2 weeks, causing:
↓ Vital capacity (VC) by 45% and ↓ FRC by 25%
These effects are seen most significantly in upper abdominal and thoracic operations.

SCC pp 65–67

Q 7.   What is measured using a spirometer?

A 7. Lung volumes can be measured directly by spirometry and vary depending on age, sex, and size (height being a closer correlate than weight) (*Fig. 2.1*).

Definitions:

■ Total lung capacity (TLC = 4.2–6 l): this is the volume of air in the lungs at the end of a maximal inspiration.

$$TLC = IRV + ERV + V_t + RV$$
$$= VC + RV$$

■ Tidal volume (V_t = 0.5 l): this is the volume of air inspired and expired during quiet breathing.
■ Inspiratory reserve volume (IRV = 1.9–3.3 l): this is the maximal volume of air that can be inspired above tidal (V_t) inspiration.
■ ERV = 0.7–1 l: this is the maximal volume of air that can be expelled after tidal (V_t) expiration.
■ VC = 3.1–4.8 l: this is the maximal volume of air that can be expired following a maximal inspiration i.e. V_t + IRV + ERV.

SCC pp 61–67

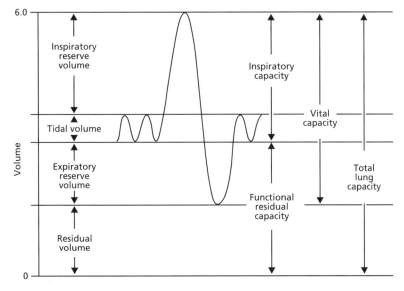

Fig. 2.1 Spirometer trace of lung volumes (Source: Pinnock, Lin and Smith (Eds): *Fundamentals of Anaesthesia* (1st Ed): GMM Ltd. London, 1999, p 413).

Q 8. What dynamic tests of respiratory function do you know?

A 8. Tests of dynamic lung performance assess forced expiration, and are measured with a spirometer.

Uses:

- Aid diagnosis
- Quantify pulmonary impairment
- Monitor the disease process
- Monitor the response to therapy

Forced expiration

- Forced vital capacity (FVC) – this is the volume of gas that can be forcibly expired after a maximal inspiration. This volume is often less than that achieved by measurement from slow expiration, due to compression of the intra-thoracic airways.
- Forced expiratory volume (FEV$_1$) – this is the volume of the vital capacity breath expired in the first second.

The FEV$_1$/FVC ratio can be used to help distinguish obstructive from restrictive limitation to expired airflow. Normally the FEV$_1$/FVC ratio is 0.8–0.9.

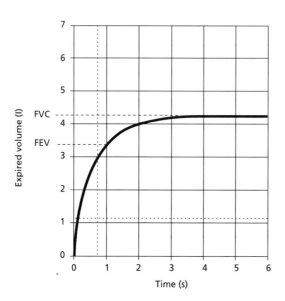

Fig. 2.2 Lung function tests (Source: Pinnock, Lin and Smith (Eds): *Fundamentals of Anaesthesia* (1st Ed): GMM Ltd. London, 1999, p 415).

1. In restrictive conditions both the FEV_1 and FVC are reduced but the ratio is typically normal or increased e.g. pulmonary conditions such as fibrosis or chest wall restrictions such as kyphoscoliosis or flail chest. This is because the vital capacity is 'restricted' i.e. reduced to a larger degree than obstructive and the limitation is overall VC rather than the time taken to expel this volume.

2. In obstructive conditions the FEV_1 is reduced to a far greater degree than the FVC, hence the ratio is much lower e.g. asthma, emphysema or any cause of obstruction such as foreign object or paralysis of the vocal cords. In this case the VC is less reduced but is 'obstructed' from being expelled by the narrowed airways (*Table 2.3*).

Table 2.3 The variation in dynamic lung function tests in obstructive and restrictive conditions

	FEV_1	FVC	Ratio
Restrictive	↓↓	↓↓	Normal or ↑
Obstructive	↓↓↓	↓	↓

Peak expiratory flow rate (PEFR)

This is used in obstructive airway conditions to assess treatment effects and reversibility. It is measured with a peak flow meter (the best of at least three attempts is the value recorded).

PEFR is reduced with:

- Asthma
- COPD
- Upper airway obstruction
- Tracheal stenosis
- Poor expiratory effort e.g. musculoskeletal problems affecting the chest wall

SCC pp 61–67

Q 9. What is meant by respiratory compliance?

A 9. Compliance is the change in volume caused by a unit change in pressure:

$$\text{Compliance} = \frac{\text{change in volume}}{\text{change in pressure}} \quad \frac{L}{kPa}$$

This measurement gives an indication of distensability of the lungs, and therefore the amount of work needed to expand them during inspiration. Compliance curves form a characteristic sigmoid-shape with increasing pressure (*Fig. 2.3*). The slope of the line gives the measure of compliance. The steeper the slope of this line the greater the compliance, so less pressure is required to produce a unit rise in volume or alternatively more volume can be inspired for unit change in pressure.

Respiratory compliance consists of chest wall and lung compliance. The tendency of the lungs to collapse by elastic recoil is countered by the tendency of the thoracic cage (chest wall) to expand outwards. The normal resting lung volume (FRC) is the equilibrium between these two opposing forces. Both lung and chest wall compliance are 200 ml/cmH$_2$O. Total respiratory compliance is a sum of the reciprocal of these two values and is usually about 100 ml/cmH$_2$O.

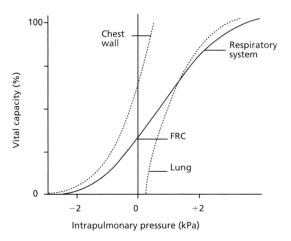

Fig. 2.3 Lung and chest wall compliance (Source: Pinnock, Lin and Smith (Eds) *Fundamentals of Anaesthesia* (1st Ed): GMM Ltd. London, 1999, p 417).

Factors decreasing compliance:

■ Extremes of lung volume (at low lung volumes there is collapse of small airways and alveoli and at high lung volumes the elastic fibres of the lung are fully stretched and large pressures are required to further increase volume)
■ Extremes of age
■ Supine posture
■ Pregnancy (because of diaphragmatic splinting)
■ ARDS
■ Pulmonary oedema/fibrosis
■ Ankalosing spondylitis
■ Kyphoscoliosis

Ventilation of patients with decreased lung compliance leads to large increases in airway pressure per unit change in volume. This risks barotrauma, damaging the lungs and further reducing the compliance.

Dynamic compliance is measured during gas flow and forms a characteristic loop. This is caused by the increased effort needed during inspiration to overcome the elastic forces resisting lung expansion. Normal expiration is a passive process driven by the stored energy from inspiration. The difference between the curves is termed hysteresis (*Fig. 2.4*).

SCC pp 62–64

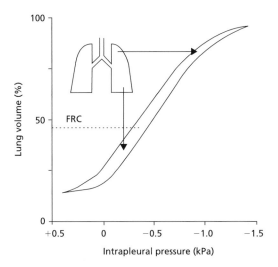

Fig. 2.4 Compliance during spontaneous ventilation (Source: Pinnock, Lin and Smith (Eds): *Fundamentals of Anaesthesia* (1st Ed): GMM Ltd. London, 1999, p 419).

Q 10. How do ventilation and perfusion vary with spontaneous and mechanical ventilation? What do you understand by the terms 'shunt' and 'dead space'?

A 10. Distribution of ventilation is uneven during the respiratory cycle. During spontaneous respiration, the majority of inspired gas passes to the lower (dependent) parts of the lung. This is because there is more negative pressure generated at the base than at the apex, favouring greater expansion. Blood flow is also greater at the base of the lung, owing to the increased hydrostatic pressure. Thus during spontaneous respiration there is good matching of ventilation (V) and perfusion (Q). Ventilation increases at a slower rate to perfusion down the lung, with the best matching of V/Q at the level of the 3rd to 4th ribs. Matching of ventilation to perfusion prevents the development of hypoxaemia, which may result from:

- Shunt – perfused areas with inadequate ventilation
- Dead space – ventilated areas with inadequate perfusion

The situation is reversed during mechanical (positive pressure) ventilation where preferential ventilation tends towards the upper (non-dependent) areas of the lung. This decreases the dependent lung volume and increases V/Q mismatch, leading to arterial hypoxaemia.

The lung has a mechanism whereby it can improve matching of V/Q by diverting blood away from area with poor ventilation. This is termed as HPV and results in decreasing the amount of shunted blood, thereby improving arterial hypoxaemia.

■ Hypoxaemia that occurs as a result of shunt cannot be improved by increasing the oxygen concentration.
■ General anaesthetics obliterate HPV and this is one reason why supplemental oxygen is required in patients during and after anaesthesia.

SCC p 65

SCC p 65

Q 11. How would you go about interpreting arterial blood gas (ABG) analysis?

A 11. Normal values:

pH	7.35–7.45
PCO_2	4.4–5.8 kPa (33–44 mmHg)
PO_2	10.0–13.3 kPa (75–100 mmHg)
SBC/HCO_3	20–30 mmol/l
ABE/SBE	−2.5 to +2.5 mmol/l
SAT	95–98 %

Check individual departmental values for normal range.

Definition of terms used:

pH – Negative logarithm (base$_{10}$) of the H^+ content in blood. The pH is inversely proportional to the blood H^+ concentration; therefore, as pH decreases so H^+ concentration rises, for example:

pH	H^+ concentration (nmol/l)
7.0	100
7.2	63
7.4	40
7.6	25

Standard bicarbonate (SBC) – It is the measure of plasma bicarbonate corrected to a PCO_2 of 5.3 kPa, removing the influence of respiratory effects on pH.

Actual base excess (ABE) – It is an *in vitro* measurement of metabolic acidosis (−ve) or alkalosis (+ve). PCO_2 is corrected to 5.3 kPa, therefore this represents the non-respiratory components only.

Standard base excess (SBE) – It is an *in vivo* assessment of acid-base balance since it adjusts for the buffering of haemoglobin and plasma proteins in whole blood compared with interstitial fluid.

Temperature has a significant effect on the results of arterial blood gas (ABG) analysis.

- Decreasing temperature decreases pH (normal pH at 27°C is 7.25)
- Decreasing temperature decreases PO_2

Therefore:

1. It is essential to key the correct body temperature into the blood gas analyser when processing samples
2. Samples should be analysed as soon as possible after they have been taken to improve the accuracy of the results

Acid-base disturbances:

Acidosis	pH < 7.35
Alkalosis	pH > 7.45

Primary change in $PaCO_2$ is respiratory
Primary change in HCO_3^- is metabolic (non-respiratory)

These changes can either be:

- Uncompensated – The pH deficit remains uncorrected
- Partially compensated – The pH is returned towards normal
- Fully compensated – The pH is returned to normal

Overcorrection is not usually possible; therefore a patient with metabolic acidosis cannot become alkalotic by compensation unless there is a compounding factor present to account for it e.g. mechanical ventilation.

Interpretation of results:

- Look at the pH – Is this alkalosis or acidosis?
- Look at the PCO_2 – Is this primarily respiratory?
- Look at the SBC – Is this primarily metabolic?

The primary disturbance is that which explains the observed pH.

- Look at the base excess is there compensation?
- Other information obtained from the ABG analysis can give further clues:
  — Is there anaemia?
  — Is there hypoxaemia?
  — Is there hyperglycaemia?
  — Is the lactate elevated?

There are often other clues from the history and clinical examination. There may be a mixed picture of respiratory and metabolic compromise, compounding the effects of the original deficit.

SCC pp 66–75

Q 12. How would you classify hypoxia?

A 12. Hypoxia is reduced oxygen delivery to the tissues of the body:

$$DO_2 = CO \% [(Hb \% {}^{Sat}/_{100} \% 1.34) + (PaO_2 \% 0.003)]$$

where, DO_2 is the oxygen delivery; CO is the cardiac output; $Hb \% {}^{Sat}/_{100} \% 1.34$ represents the amount of oxygen carried by haemoglobin in the blood (1.34 is a calculation constant); $PaO_2 \% 0.003$ represents the amount of oxygen dissolved in blood, and is usually negligible compared to that combined with haemoglobin.

There are several types of hypoxia depending on where the reduction in oxygen delivery occurs.

Hypoxic hypoxia
This results in $\downarrow$ Sat and $\downarrow PaO_2$ and is caused by:

- Low oxygen concentration of the inspired gas mixture e.g. at altitude
- Hypoventilation e.g. atelectasis and airway collapse, airway obstruction, drugs (opioids and anaesthetic agents), central depression of ventilation
- Diffusion failure between the alveolus and capillary e.g. pulmonary oedema and fibrosis or pneumonia
- Ventilation/perfusion imbalance e.g. ARDS
- Shunting of blood from the venous to arterial circulation e.g. cyanotic heart disease

Anaemic hypoxia
This is the result of low Hb which may be caused by:

■ ↓ Red blood corpuscle (RBC) from ↓ production, blood loss or ↑ destruction
■ ↓ Hb per RBC e.g. hypochromic anaemia of iron deficiency
■ Abnormal forms of Hb e.g. sickle cell disease
■ Reduced binding of oxygen to Hb e.g. carbon monoxide poisoning

At rest, anaemic hypoxia is not usually a problem, unless the patient has co-existing ischaemic heart disease. During exercise, there can be severe limitation.

Stagnant hypoxia
This is due to a low cardiac output and causes high oxygen extraction leading to lower venous oxygen content. There is also decreased removal of waste products of metabolism leading to the accumulation of lactate (metabolic acidosis).

Histotoxic hypoxia
Here the delivery of oxygen to the tissues is adequate but they are unable to utilise it e.g. cyanide poisoning.

SCC pp 76–78

Q 13. Which patients are at risk of post-operative hypoxaemia? What methods are available to deliver oxygen to a spontaneously breathing patient after surgery?

A 13. Hypoxaemia can occur with any patient after surgery. Some groups of patients are at higher risk, and should receive prolonged oxygen therapy (at least 72 hours):

■ Ischaemic heart disease
■ Anaemia
■ Major abdominal (esp. upper gastrointestinal tract (GIT)) and thoracic operations
■ Hypotension/low CO (it is important to treat the cause)
■ Hypothermia
■ Obese patients ⎫
■ Hyperthermia/sepsis ⎬ these have an increased oxygen
■ Shivering ⎭ demand

Variable performance oxygen delivery systems

The oxygen concentration delivered to the patient is not constant and depends on the minute volume (MV), or more specifically the peak inspiratory flow rate (PIFR). As the PIFR increases more air will be entrained from the surroundings and the oxygen concentration delivered to the patient will decrease, unless the oxygen flow rate is increased. The following are two examples of systems commonly used after surgery (Table 2.4):

Table 2.4 The different systems for delivering variable concentrations of oxygen

Hudson mask		Nasal specs	
O_2 flow (l/min)	O_2 conc. (%)	O_2 flow (l/min)	O_2 conc. (%)
2	24–38	1	25–29
4	35–45	2	29–35
6	51–61	4	32–39
8	57–67		
10	61–73		

Fixed-performance oxygen delivery systems (Venturi masks)

These deliver a constant oxygen concentration independent of the patient's respiratory pattern (MV and PIFR). The oxygen supply entrains air at a fixed rate via a jet built into the mask. The total flow rate is therefore higher than the PIFR and dilution of the oxygen supply does not occur. The jet entrainment devices are coloured coded and higher flow rates must be dialled when increased oxygen concentrations are required (Table 2.5).

Table 2.5 The system for delivering a known concentration of oxygen

Colour code	O_2 supply flow rate (l/min)	Delivered O_2 conc. (%)
White	4	28
Yellow	8	35
Red	10	40
Green	15	60

SCC pp 76–78

Q 14. How would you classify respiratory failure, and what are the signs?

A 14. Respiratory failure occurs when the PaO_2 and $PaCO_2$ can no longer be maintained within normal limits. If untreated this leads on to cellular hypoxaemia and acidosis by decreasing the capacity for gaseous exchange. Respiratory failure may be split up into two types, depending on the CO_2 concentration present in blood. Patients may progress from one type to the other:

Type I: ↓ PaO_2 with normal or ↓ $PaCO_2$ (there may be respiratory alkalosis)

- Pulmonary embolism
- Fibrosing alveolitis
- Pneumonia ⎫
- Asthma ⎬ when severe, these conditions may be associated with Type II failure
- Early ARDS ⎭

Type II: Ventilatory Failure

↓ PaO_2 with ↑ $PaCO_2$ (respiratory acidosis)

- Mechanical obstruction to the airway e.g. vomit, blood, foreign body or tumour
- Obstructive airways disease e.g. COPD, severe asthma
- Advanced ARDS
- Severe pneumonia
- Neuromuscular disorders e.g. cervical cord injury, polio, Guillain Barré, motor neurone disease
- Chest wall deformities e.g. chest trauma (flail chest), ankalosing spondylitis, kyphoscoliosis
- Central depression of respiratory drive e.g. drugs (especially sedatives), head injury, brain tumours

Signs of respiratory failure

- Tachypnoea
- Dyspnoea
- Tachycardia
- The use of accessory muscles of respiration
    — intercostal recession
    — subcostal recession
    — tracheal tug

- Inability to speak in sentences (leading on to total inability to speak)
- Impaired consciousness (this is a grave sign)
- Cyanosis is a blue/purple discolouration of the skin caused by the presence of deoxyhaemoglobin (in amounts >5 g/dl). This is a notoriously unreliable sign, particularly in areas with poor or artificial lighting. It is possible to observe:
  — Cyanosis without hypoxia (polycythaemia)
  — Hypoxia without cyanosis (anaemia)

SCC pp 79–80

Q 15. What are the indications for intubation and mechanical ventilation?

A 15. Positive pressure ventilation may be required for signs of respiratory failure. The decision whether to institute ventilatory support should be taken by a senior clinician, and is based on several factors, including:

- The pre-morbid health status of the patient is an important index of survivability following admission to the intensive care unit (ICU).
- There should be potential reversibility of the admitting condition.

Indications for mechanical ventilation

Inadequate ventilation:

- Apnoea
- RR > 35/min   (Normal range is 12–20/min for adults)
- VC < 15 ml/kg   (Normal range is 65–75 ml/kg)
- TV < 5 ml/kg   (Normal range is 5–7 ml/kg)
- $PaCO_2 > 8$ kPa   (This depends on the patients normal $PaCO_2$)

Inadequate oxygenation:

- $PaO_2 < 8$ kPa   (Breathing > 60% oxygen)

Specific surgical indications:
Head injury – If this results in an unprotected airway, there is an increased risk of gastric aspiration with the development of chemical pneumonitis. Other indications are a lowered Glasgow coma score (GCS) (this is usually taken as below 8) or if there are symptoms and signs of raised intracranial pressure (in order to control the $PaCO_2$).

Chest injury – This may be required with a flail chest, the dyskinetic segment contributing little to the efficiency of ventilation. There may be a pneumothorax, which should be drained prior to intubation and positive pressure ventilation. Undrained pneumothoraces have the potential to tamponade with intermittent positive pressure ventilation (IPPV). The presence of a pulmonary contusion may reduce the efficiency of gas exchange and require ventilation.

Facial trauma – Bleeding into the airway makes breathing laboured and may obstruct the airway completely. Swallowed blood is extremely emetogenic and may lead to aspiration of stomach contents. There may be disruption of the airway architecture resulting in partial or complete airway compromise. There may also be an associated head injury (or neck injury).

High spinal injury – Patients with injuries to the spinal cord below the level of C5 may have relatively little in the way of respiratory compromise, as the diaphragm continues to provide much of the inspiratory excursion required. Above this, however there will be respiratory difficulties since the phrenic nerve arises from C3, 4, 5. There may also be potential respiratory compromise from gastric aspiration, or any associated head injury or facial trauma described above.

Burns – Circumferential burns to the neck or the chest need prompt intubation and ventilation since severe respiratory compromise can occur. The airway may be obstructed and respiratory excursion may be severely limited, requiring simultaneous escharotomy. Smoke or steam inhalation requires intubation as soon as possible to prevent subsequent airway compromise. The only signs may be the presence of soot on the nose or mouth.

The trachea should be intubated in the following circumstances:

- Risk of gastric aspiration in the unprotected airway (to protect the lower airway)
- Upper airway obstruction
- To facilitate the use of positive pressure ventilation

SCC pp 80–87

Respiratory System

Answers

Q 16. What are the effects of mechanical ventilation?

A 16. The principle for gas flow with IPPV is the same as for spontaneous ventilation. Gas flows down a pressure gradient from the mouth to the alveoli. The difference, however, lies in that the proximal driving pressure is positive rather than atmospheric, and the distal pressure is zero rather than negative. Work is still done to expand the lung and chest wall and this is stored and used to drive expiration, which is passive. IPPV effects many body systems:

Respiratory

- FRC is recovered, improving the efficiency of ventilation. The inspired oxygen concentration can be adjusted to optimise oxygenation, and CO_2 removal is improved in patients with respiratory failure.
- Lung water can be reduced, further improving oxygenation
- The high pressures sometimes needed to expand the lung can cause damage due to barotrauma, leading to pneumothorax formation. This is especially true when the respiratory compliance is reduced e.g. with ARDS. Subsequent ventilation with drained pneumothoraces can be difficult and inefficient, due to air leaks.
- Reduction of HPV, with resultant increased mismatching of ventilation

Cardiovascular
There is an overall reduction in BP and CO:

- Reduced pre-load ($\downarrow$ venous return to the right ventricle) due to loss of negative pressure intra-thoracic pump
- Increased pulmonary vascular resistance (PVR) – this leads initially to right ventricular dilatation resulting in inadequate left ventricular filling (because of volume increase in RV)
- Sedation reduces the arterial BP
- Correction of hypoxia, hypercarbia and acidosis decreases endogenous catecholamine drive on the cardiovascular system (CVS)

Renal

- Decreased cardiac output results in:
  — $\downarrow$ Renal blood flow
  — $\downarrow$ Renal perfusion pressure

— ↓ Glomerular filtration rate

— ↓ Urine output

Cerebral

- Increased intra-thoracic pressure is transmitted through the venous system to ↑ intra-cranial pressure (ICP)
- Conversely reduction of CO_2 by ventilation reduces cerebral blood volume thereby ↓ ICP

Metabolic

- Titration of $PaCO_2$ can be used to compensate for acid-base disturbances

SCC pp 80–87

Q 17. What modes of mechanical ventilation do you know? Which of these modes are used for weaning?

A 17. Controlled mandatory ventilation (CMV)

- The ventilator will deliver a set tidal volume (V_t) at a set respiratory rate (RR)
- No inspiratory effort is made by the patient
- Any attempt to breathe or cough by the patient during inspiration can result in dangerously high peak airway pressures (PAWP), leading to barotrauma
- The patient must be deeply sedated and is often paralysed

Synchronised intermittent mandatory ventilation (SIMV)

- The minute volume is composed of a mixture of mandatory V_t breaths (initiated by the ventilator) and some spontaneous breaths (initiated by the patient)
- There is co-ordination (synchronisation) between the ventilator-initiated breaths and the patient-initiated breaths, so that both are not delivered simultaneously. This prevents the high PAWP sometimes seen with CMV
- The patients may be less deeply sedated and muscle paralysis is rarely required

SIMV has a number of advantages over CMV:

- ↓ level of sedation required
- ↓ incidence of ↑ PAWP (hence ↓ incidence of barotrauma)

- ↓ mean airway pressure (MAWP) ⇒ less ↓ in CO and BP (greater haemodynamic stability)
- Better matching of ventilation and perfusion
- Easier assessment of spontaneous breathing activity
- Improved weaning from ventilation (less disuse atrophy of the respiratory muscles since spontaneous ventilation is not discouraged)

Pressure control ventilation (PCV)

CMV and SIMV are examples of volume-controlled ventilation, where a pre-set volume is delivered to the patient. PCV differs in that the pressure is set and the volume delivered to the patient will vary depending on the compliance (*see* previous section) of the lungs and the inspiratory time.

- Patients with ↓ lung compliance will receive a ↓ V_t for any set pressure
- Square wave pressure trace
- MAWP is higher for any level of PAWP
  — ↑ MAWP equates with ↑ oxygenation
- ↓ PAWP ⇒ ↓ risk of barotrauma
- RR set on ventilator
- Start with pressure of 30 cmH$_2$O to give V_t of 10–12 ml/kg (depends on lung compliance)

Pressure support ventilation (PSV)

This is sometimes referred to as pressure assisted ventilation:

- The patient triggers the ventilator to deliver a pre-set pressure to the lungs
- RR determined by the patient
- V_t depends on the level of pressure support (PS) and the lung compliance
- Set level of PS to give V_t of 10–12 ml/kg (usually 15–30 cmH$_2$O)

This mode of ventilation can be used in isolation or in conjunction with PCV or SIMV. Its main use is for weaning from ventilation, with the level of PS reduced as the mechanics of respiration improve:

- Minimal sedation needed (only to tolerate the ETT).
- Has the advantage of maintaining muscular activity, thereby minimising the risks of disuse atrophy.

SIMV and PSV are the main weaning modes. SIMV differs in that the ventilator will always give some mandatory breaths, with spontaneous breaths being 'triggered' by the patient. PSV has no mandatory breaths and 'patient-triggered' breaths makes up the entire minute volume. With both of these modes any inspiratory effort by the patient (triggering), is sensed and the ventilator is instructed to assist the breath. As weaning progresses, the level of inspiratory effort required to trigger an assisted breath is increased and the level of support is decreased, increasing the patient's contribution until they are eventually able to breathe unaided.

SCC pp 80–87

Q 18. Why is it important to maintain adequate lung volume? What methods do you know for optimising lung volume?

A 18. Manoeuvres designed to optimise lung volume aim to increase FRC by alveolar recruitment, re-expanding collapsed areas of the lung. This places the lung on a more efficient (steeper) part of the compliance curve, generating maximum volume change per unit increase in pressure. Maintaining lung volume prevents airway collapse and alveolar atelectasis, thus minimising shunt and reducing the effective dead space per breath. This reduces the work of breathing and optimises arterial oxygenation for any given inspired oxygen concentration (F_iO_2).

The F_iO_2 should be set at a level that is as low as possible to prevent hypoxaemia. The proportion of nitrogen in the lungs is important since this inert gas does not take part in gaseous exchange. Oxygen is readily absorbed from the alveoli into the capillary network leading to absorption atelectasis. A higher F_iO_2 reduces the ratio of nitrogen to oxygen, increasing this tendency to collapse.

The following methods may be employed to optimise lung volume:

- Continuous positive airways pressure (CPAP) is used during spontaneous ventilation
- Positive end expiratory pressure (PEEP) is used during ventilator delivered breaths

Typically 5–10 cmH$_2$O is used. More may be used with mechanical ventilation and patients with uncompliant lungs e.g. ARDS may require upto 15 cmH$_2$O of PEEP. Both these methods increase the risk of barotrauma and volutrauma and should be used with caution in asthmatic patients (risk of extremely high airway pressures).

■ Inverse ratio ventilation (IRV). The usual I:E ratio of 1:2 gives adequate time for expiration, which is passive. Reversing the ratio to 1:1, 2:1 or 3:1 will progressively decrease the time for expiration, which will generate AUTOPEEP. This increases the MAWP without increasing the PAWP. This improves oxygenation, without any increased risk of barotrauma. IRV requires deep sedation and paralysis since it is a very unnatural and uncomfortable mode of ventilation.

Associated effects of these manoeuvres to optimise lung volume:

■ The increased intra-thoracic pressure is transmitted via the venous system to the CNS, increasing ICP
■ The increased intra-thoracic pressure reduces venous return lowering CO and BP
■ CO$_2$ elimination is reduced resulting in respiratory acidosis

SCC pp 80–87

Q 19. What factors affect the ability to wean from mechanical ventilation?

A 19. The 'weaning' process is re-institution of independent spontaneous respiration after a period of ventilatory support. The withdrawal of artificial ventilation is achieved gradually and success depends on several factors:

Duration of mechanical ventilation – The weaning process is quicker with post-operative cases (<24 hours ventilated).

Past medical history – Respiratory and cardiovascular disease can pose a significant hurdle to rapid successful weaning.

Current medical problems – Active chest infection, significant areas of collapse or consolidation, and heart failure greatly decrease the chances of success. These conditions are relative contra-indications to active weaning.

Nutritional state and muscle power

Drugs – Residual levels of opioids, sedatives and muscle relaxants will determine the effectiveness and speed of the weaning process.

Signs of failure during weaning

- Tachypnoea and dyspnoea
- Hypoxia and hypercarbia
- Use of accessory muscles of respiration
- Exhaustion and fatigue leading to reduced conscious level

Weaning pre-conditions

- Starts only after recovery from the pathology that required ventilatory support
- Haemodynamic stability
- Optimisation of oxygen delivery to the tissues – Hb and cardiac output
- Optimisation of nutritional status to prevent muscle fatigue
- Active sepsis and pyrexia should be excluded since these increase oxygen demand and may lead to early failure
- F_iO_2 should be <0.6

Practical aspects of weaning from ventilatory support

- Weaning plan should be started as early as possible in the day – ideally after the morning ward round
- Minimise sedation and opioid analgesia – however bear in mind that pain increases oxygen demand and risk of failure
- Decrease mandatory respiratory rate delivered by the ventilator – gradually towards zero
- Decrease the pressure support level – maintaining adequate V_t
- Decrease PEEP
- When: SIMV rate $= 0$
         PS $= 10\,cmH_2O$
         PEEP $= 5\,cmH_2O$

Then the patient may be put on a T-piece ($\pm$ CPAP of $5\,cmH_2O$) for a few hours at a time, alternating with PS via the ventilator. Good clinical and ABG monitoring is required until the patient is able to maintain adequate ventilation independently. This process may take weeks to complete. There is currently no reliable predictor of successful weaning.

SCC pp 80–87

Q 20. What are the causes of airway obstruction? How may these be managed?

A 20. Airway obstruction usually occurs in the unconscious patient and may be partial or complete. It may occur anywhere from the nose or mouth down to the trachea.

There are many causes of an obstructed airway:

- Relaxation of the soft tissues (especially the tongue) in the oropharynx
- Vomit, blood or other foreign body
- Laryngospasm
- Facial trauma
- Oedema of the airway secondary to burns or smoke inhalation, infection or inflammation, and anaphylactoid reactions
- Lower airway obstruction (sub-laryngeal) is less common and associated with:
  — Pulmonary secretions and mucous plugging (common in ICU patients)
  — Thoracic trauma
  — Obstructive airways – asthma or emphysema (expiration)
  — Pulmonary oedema
  — Large pneumothorax/haemothorax

Clinical

- Complete obstruction is silent
- Partial obstruction is noisy
- There may be paradoxical (see-saw) movements of the chest and abdomen caused by uncoordinated movements of the respiratory muscles

Manoeuvres designed to keep the upper airway patent aim to achieve the 'sniffing the morning air' position with the neck flexed and head extended:

- Head tilt – avoid in trauma patients
- Chin lift
- Jaw thrust – this is the safest method for patients with suspected neck injury (in conjunction with in-line stabilisation)

These techniques may be supplemented by:

- Oropharyngeal (Guedel) airway
- Nasopharyngeal airway (not with suspected base-of-skull fracture)
- Laryngeal mask airway (LMA) – is relatively easy to insert and rests in the hypopharynx cushioned by an air-filled cuff. Although not a definitive airway, this can be used for positive pressure ventilation for short periods or in an emergency (with a variable leak around the cuff).

Definitive airway
Endo-tracheal tube:

- Nasal is more comfortable and therefore requires less sedation
- Oral makes suctioning and fibreoptic examination of the lower airway easier

Tracheostomy:

- Mini-tracheostomy – usually as an emergency procedure for ventilation or expectoration and suctioning of excessive lower airway secretions. It is not suitable for prolonged ventilation since the narrow bore of the tube does not allow adequate CO_2 clearance.
- Percutaneous – using a Seldinger technique. A fibreoptic scope may also be used to aid visualisation.
- Surgical

Indications for a definitive airway

- Protection of the lower airway from aspiration by food, blood, secretions or vomit (any patient with a GCS $<$ 8 will need airway protection)
- Facilitation of positive pressure ventilation
- By-passing any upper airway obstruction
- Allows regular suction of the lower airway and aspiration of samples for culture

SCC pp 87–91

Q 21. **What are the principle causes of ARDS? What clinical findings make up the diagnosis?**

A 21. ARDS is the pulmonary component of the systemic inflammatory response syndrome (SIRS).

Direct (pulmonary) causes

- Contusion from blunt trauma
- Aspiration of stomach contents
- Near drowning
- Infection
- Smoke or toxic inhalation

Indirect (extra-pulmonary) causes

- Sepsis
- Major trauma
- Embolic episodes (thrombotic, fat or amniotic)
- Pancreatitis
- Massive blood transfusion
- Severe or prolonged haemorrhage/hypotension
- Disseminated intravascular coagulopathy (DIC)
- Cardio-pulmonary bypass

The incidence varies from 3 to 6 per 10^5 in the UK, upto 80 per 10^5 of the population in the USA. This variability has much to do with differences in diagnosis between the two countries, which led to a consensus conference formulating the following criteria:

- There must be a known precipitating cause
- The onset of symptoms must be acute
- There must be hypoxia refractory to oxygen therapy
- There must be new bilateral, fluffy infiltrates on the CXR (this sign may lag behind the clinical picture by 12–24 hours)
- There must be no cardiac failure or fluid overload (this is to exclude these causes of the typical CXR appearance in ARDS, and is taken as a PAWP of <18 mmHg)

The severity of the hypoxic insult can be quantified into acute lung injury (ALI) or ARDS depending on the fraction of inspired oxygen that the subject is breathing:

- In ALI the $PaO_2:F_IO_2$ ratio is <40 kPa (300 mmHg)
- In ARDS the $PaO_2:F_IO_2$ ratio is <27 kPa (200 mmHg)

The following are associated clinical findings (but are not included as diagnostic criteria):

- The need for mechanical ventilation
- Low lung compliance

SCC pp 91–96

Q 22. **Describe the pathophysiological processes responsible for ARDS? What is the prognosis?**

A 22. The pathophysiology of ARDS revolves around the protective inflammatory response to invasion by chemical or infective toxins. This response is subject to positive feedback resulting in an uncontrolled and damaging series of events that result in the clinical findings of ARDS.

In the early stages (within 24 hours of the precipitating event) there is neutrophil activation leading to the release of inflammatory mediators such as cytokines, tumour necrosis factor (TNF), platelet activating factor (PAF), interleukin (IL1 and IL6) and proteases. These inflammatory mediators cause direct capillary endothelial cell damage resulting in increased capillary permeability. This leads to a 'leakage' of protein rich exudate, which fills the alveoli. The fluid filled alveoli do not take part in gaseous exchange resulting in shunt formation and hypoxaemia. As the fluid is reabsorbed there is atelectic collapse of the affected alveoli with the resulting loss of functional lung units. Arterial hypoxaemia is compounded by direct damage to lung parenchyma by the inflammatory mediators.

The late stages of ARDS are characterised by fibroblast proliferation into the affected lung units, resulting in fibrosis and collagen deposition. This leads to microvascular obliteration compounding the ventilation/perfusion mismatch. Eventually the patient may develop a clinical picture similar to fibrosing alveolitis, with restrictive lung disease symptoms.

The disease process is not uniform within the lung, with some areas being spared and capable of gas exchange.

Prognosis
This is extremely variable and the mortality is increased by:

■ Increasing age
■ Significant past medical history – especially renal or hepatic failure

- Precipitating cause – sepsis has the highest mortality and polytrauma (provided the patient survives the initial event) has the lowest
- Associated complications increase morbidity and can worsen mortality

Early deaths are often related to the precipitating cause, late deaths are frequently associated with multi-organ failure (MOF). Many survivors have little or no residual problems; others will have a range of disability from a reduced exercise tolerance to symptoms and signs of fibrotic lung disease.

SCC pp 91–96

Q 23. **What are the objectives for respiratory support in a patient with ARDS? What mechanisms are there to maintain adequate oxygenation?**

A 23. The aim is to achieve reasonable levels of oxygenation and CO_2 removal without any further damage to the lungs. This may require a compromise between adequate ventilation and protection of the healthy lung. This may be achieved by:

- Permissible hypercapnia to $PaCO_2$ of 10–15 kPa (if no signs of acidosis of cerebral oedema)
- Acceptable hypoxaemia to PaO_2 of 8 kPa (if no signs of ischaemia)

Methods of ventilatory support
Collapsed areas of the lung may be expanded by alveolar recruitment manoeuvres designed to increase the FRC, thereby improving oxygenation:

- CPAP (5–10 cmH$_2$O) can be used in spontaneously breathing patients in the early stages of the disease, and may be administered via a nasal or facemask. It is seldom effective for long-term therapy and is usually a holding measure.
- PEEP (10–15 cmH$_2$O) can be used during mechanical ventilation but is associated with haemodynamic instability.

Conventional volume-controlled ventilation with tidal volumes of 10–12 ml/kg can cause barotrauma and volutrauma to the healthy areas of the lung. These can be avoided by the following manoeuvres:

PCV – This generates a characteristic square waveform so optimising MAWP without increasing (PAWP). The upper pressure is limited to that set on the ventilator. This is usually set to 30–40 cmH$_2$O.

IRV – Normal inspiratory (I) to expiratory (E) ratio is 1:2, but this can lead to high inflation pressures because of the relatively short inspiratory time and the stiff lungs. The I:E ratio may be prolonged to 1:1, 2:1 or 3:1. This will further optimise the MAWP, so improving oxygenation for any given PAWP. There are several problems associated with these methods of ventilation:

- Haemodynamic instability
- Decrease in CO$_2$ elimination leading to further hypercapnia
- Deep sedation and paralysis are required since this is a very unnatural and uncomfortable mode of ventilation.

Resistant hypoxaemia may benefit from improved matching of ventilation (V) and perfusion (Q) by changing the position of the patient:

- Prone ventilation (usually for 4–8 hours at a time). This strategy aims to decrease the collapse seen in the dependant areas of the lung by reducing the time that the patient spends in one position. Gradually the dependent areas in the new position will collapse and contribute towards hypoxaemia, and the position will need to be changed again. This can be very labour intensive for the nursing staff.
- Ventilation on a rotating bed. By continuously moving the patient through 90° areas of the lung will only become dependent transiently and therefore reduce the incidence of collapse.

Both of these manoeuvres are made more hazardous by the use of multiple infusion lines or haemofiltration.

Prostacyclin and nitric oxide (NO) also known as endothelium derived relaxant factor (EDRF). When delivered via a specialised circuit these agents selectively vasodilate the pulmonary vascular beds that are adequately ventilated, thus improving V/Q matching and improving hypoxaemia.

SCC pp 91–96

Respiratory System

Answers

Q 1. **What are the indications for a computed tomography (CT) scan following a head injury?**

A 1. With the advent of high-speed spiral scanners, computed tomography (CT) scans are used liberally in the management of head injury. General guidelines for a CT scan are:

- Deterioration in conscious level as assessed by the Glasgow coma score (GCS) or development of pupillary signs
- Development of focal neurological signs
- Skull fracture
- The patient remains confused or in a state of unconsciousness
- The patient is difficult to assess e.g. alcohol
- Penetrating injury

SCC pp 99–107

Q 2. **What type of injuries are possible to blood vessels and what are their sequelae?**

A 2. Both arteries and veins can be injured by either transection (incomplete or complete), laceration or closed injuries.

Incomplete transection:

- Pulsatile haematoma
- Delayed haemorrhage
- False aneurysm
- Rupture
- Thrombosis and embolism
- Arteriovenous fistula

Complete transection:

- Contraction
- Retraction
- Haematoma
- Distal ischaemia
- Pulse deficit

Complicated laceration with loss of tissue:

The extent of injury is often greater than the defect. Patches are often required

- Distal thrombosis
- Distal ischaemia
- Haematoma (pulsatile)
- False aneurysm

Closed injury:

- Thrombosis
- Intimal flap or tear
- Dissection
- Occlusion
- Spasm

SCC pp 146–151

Q 3. **What are the causes of raised intracranial pressure (ICP) after head injury?**

A 3. The causes of raised intracranial pressure (ICP) after head injury are:

- Haematoma
- Focal cerebral oedema (contusion or haematoma)
- Diffuse oedema
- Diffuse brain swelling
- Cerebrospinal fluid (CSF) obstruction (rare)

Raised intracranial pressure (ICP) jeopardises cerebral perfusion (Cerebral perfusion pressure (CPP) = Mean arterial pressure (MAP) − ICP).

SCC pp 99–107

Q 4. **What are the indications for urgent surgical exploration in thoracic trauma?**

A 4. Thoracic trauma can result in either intrathoracic injury or intra-abdominal injury, and therefore surgical exploration can be either thoracotomy or laparotomy (*Table 3.1*).

Table 3.1 Indications for surgical exploration in thoracic trauma

Indications for thoracotomy	
Initial drainage >1500 ml	Obvious intra-abdominal injury
Drainage >500 ml for 3 or more hours	Positive DPL
Signs of occult haemorrhage with no other injury	Obvious diaphragmatic injury
Massive air leak	Suspected penetrating diaphragmatic injury
Praecordial penetrating injury	
Ruptured aorta	
Massive chest wall defect	

SCC pp 146–151

Q 5. **How do you decide how much fluid to give a patient with major burns?**

A 5. Fluid replacement with either colloid or crystalloid should be instigated as soon after a major burn as possible, and should be in line with one of the recommended regimens: e.g. Parkland (ATLS®).

Weight (kg) × % Burn surface area × (2 to 4)

This replacement is from the time of the burn and represents fluid load for the first 24 hours.

SCC pp 151–157

Q 6. **How do you diagnose and treat fat embolism syndrome (FES)?**

A 6. **Signs and symptoms**
The signs and symptoms of fat embolism syndrome (FES) can be divided into respiratory, central nervous system (CNS) and other (*Table 3.2*).

Table 3.2 Signs and Symptoms of FES

Respiratory	*CNS*	*Other*
Dyspnoea	Anxiety	Petechial rash
Tachypnoea	Irritation	Retinal haemorrhages
Hypoxaemia*	Confusion	Tachycardia
CXR – Bilateral infiltrates	Convulsions	Fever
Adult respiratory distress syndrome (ARDS)	CT – Cerebral oedema	

* Hypoxaemia can persist up to 14 days

Diagnosis

Diagnosis is made based on the criteria of Gurd and Wilson (*Table 3.3*). One major and four minor criteria are required, including fat macroglobulinaemia ($>8\,\mu m$).

Table 3.3 Gurd and Wilson's Diagnostic Criteria for FES

Major	*Minor*	*Laboratory*
Petechial rash on upper anterior body	Tachycardia	Acute $\downarrow$ haemoglobin
Respiratory symptoms, signs or X-ray changes	Pyrexia	Sudden thrombocytopenia
Cerebral signs unrelated to head injury	Retinal changes	$\uparrow$ Erythrocyte sedimentation rate (ESR)
	Renal changes	Fat macroglobulinaemia
	Jaundice	

Source: Gurd AR, Wilson RI. *J Bone Joint Surg* 1974: 58; 408–416

Treatment

The mainstay of treatment of FES is supportive. Respiratory support (oxygen, continuous positive airway pressure (CPAP), intermittent positive pressure ventilation (IPPV)), cardiovascular support (maintenance of intravascular volume and oxygen delivery which may require inotropes), CNS support (control ICP) and musculoskeletal support by immobilisation of fractures.

SCC pp 158–160

Other Systems and Multisystem Failure

Answers

Q 7. What features of burn injuries would make you suspect an inhalational injury and how would you manage it?

A 7. Inhalational injury is characterised by evidence of laryngeal oedema (cough, stridor, hoarse voice, carbon deposits around mouth).

Smoke inhalation is investigated by measurement of carboxyhaemoglobin levels, arterial blood gases and fibreoptic bronchoscopy to assess the upper airway.

Treatment is principally of respiratory support; intubate and 100% oxygen, CPAP and positive end expiratory pressure (PEEP), regular bronchodilators and chest physiotherapy.

Complications of smoke inhalation include airway compromise, oedema and obstruction, which is an emergency. Other complications include airway irritation leading to bronchospasm and mucus production, decreased lung compliance and increased lung lymph production.

SCC pp 151–157

Q 8. How would you assess the severity of a head injury?

A 8. First priorities are to stabilise circulation and respiration (i.e. oxygenation, ventilation and perfusion). This prevents secondary damage.

Assessment is by the GCS – not just at one point in time but also trends in the GCS.

History of the injury including duration of amnesia (both antegrade and retrograde), mechanism of injury, and AMPLE (advanced trauma life support – ATLS®) history.

Examination including full secondary survey, treatment of concomitant injuries.

Radiological investigations including skull X-ray and CT scan as indicated.

ICP monitoring is necessary in severe head injuries.

SCC pp 99–107

Q 9. **What are the causes of massive haemoptysis and how would you manage a patient with it?**

A 9. Massive haemoptysis accounts for only 1.5% of all haemoptysis. Any bleeding originating from the bronchial arteries may cause life-threatening haemoptysis because of the high pressure in the bronchial arteries. The overall mortality rate attributed to massive haemoptysis is largely influenced by malignant aetiologies and by the rate of bleeding.

Causes include neoplasm, bronchiectasis, infections, vascular, vasculitis but others also occur.

Establish the source of the bleeding

- Haemorrhagic sites from the nasopharynx or the gastrointestinal tract should be excluded.
- Majority of haemoptysis prevalence originates from the bronchial arteries (90%).
- Pulmonary arteries may be the cause in only 5%.
- Bleeding tends to be more significant when coming from the bronchial arteries because of high systemic pressure.

Clinical history
Salient points in the history include:

- Anticoagulant therapy or coagulopathies may cause haemoptysis in patients with no prior history of lung diseases or haemoptysis.
- Pulmonary tuberculosis may lead to haemoptysis caused by erosion of blood vessels.
- Prior diagnosis of cavitary diseases such as tuberculosis, sarcoidosis, or chronic obstructive pulmonary diseases.
- Bronchogenic carcinoma should be high in the list among smokers >40 years of age.
- Bronchial adenoma, vascular anomalies, and aspiration of foreign bodies are very common causes of haemoptysis among children.
- Patients with congestive heart failure secondary to mitral stenosis are at risk for haemoptysis.
- A history of deep vein thrombosis may lead to pulmonary infarct and embolism.

- Febrile conditions with pulmonary infections (lung abscess, necrotising pneumonia) may be complicated by massive haemoptysis.

Physical examination

- The presence of stridor or wheezing should raise the suspicion of tracheolaryngeal tumours or foreign body.
- Concomitant haematuria suggests a diagnosis of Goodpasture's syndrome.
- Clubbing may be a sign of lung carcinoma or bronchiectasis.

Diagnostic studies

- Sputum examination – Sputum should be examined for the presence of bacteria (Gram stain and acid-fast bacillus). A smear for cytology should be done if the patient is >40 years of age and a smoker. A specimen should also be obtained for culture, especially for mycobacterium and fungus.
- Chest radiography – May identify lung parenchymal pathologies (e.g. tumours).
- Bronchoscopy – Rigid bronchoscopy is recommended in the event of massive haemoptysis because of its greater suctioning ability and maintenance of airway patency. Failure to visualise the upper lobes or peripheral lesions remains a major limitation with rigid bronchoscope. Instillation of a vasoactive drug directly into the bleeding bronchus through the bronchoscope channel may stop the haemorrhage.
- CT – CT may demonstrate lesions that may not be visible in the chest radiograph, such as bronchiectasis or small bronchial carcinoma. When performed with contrast material, CT may detect thoracic aneurysm or arteriovenous malformations.

Management

- Resuscitation
- Vital signs and oxygen saturation should be monitored in the intensive therapy unit (ITU).
- Blood investigations including full blood count, arterial blood gas, coagulation profile, electrolytes, type and cross-match (minimum of 6 units of packed red cells), renal and liver function tests.

- Intubation is necessary for life-threatening haemoptysis, hypovolemic shock, worsening hypoxemia in spite of supplemental oxygen or an elevated CO_2 concentration.
- Surgery and other invasive methods:
  - Surgery remains the procedure of choice in the treatment of massive haemoptysis caused by leaky aortic aneurysm, arteriovenous malformations, iatrogenic pulmonary rupture, chest injuries, and bronchial adenoma.
- Endobronchial tamponade (occluding the bleeding bronchus with a balloon catheter). The insertion of these catheters necessitates the use of a rigid or flexible bronchoscope.
- Bronchial artery embolisation (BAE) is now considered the most effective non-surgical treatment in massive haemoptysis because of immediate and long-term results. Selective angiography should be performed initially to locate the bleeding bronchial artery before injection.
- Conservative management. Invasive therapeutic measures are not indicated in the control of haemoptysis caused by anticoagulant therapy or blood dyscrasia. These conditions can be treated by appropriate medical therapy.

Q 10. How would you manage a patient with acute hepatic failure (AHF)?

A 10. The aims of management of acute hepatic failure (AHF) are the prevention of complications, namely infection, cerebral oedema and multiple organ failure and to optimise conditions for hepatic regeneration. The other principle is the identification of potential transplant recipients. Early transfer to a specialist unit is recommended. The mainstay is supportive therapy.

Precipitating factors for AHF should be reversed where possible (GI bleed, renal failure). Oral lactulose should be administered and dietary protein decreased.

Other systems should be supported; fluid replacement – 5% dextrose is fluid of choice, inotropes for cardiovascular system (CVS), mechanical ventilation $\pm$ PEEP for RS and Mannitol 0.5 g/kg $\pm$ Frusemide for cerebral oedema.

- Infection should be controlled, considering selective decontamination of the gut with neomycin.

- Support other systems.
- Liver assist devices are undergoing studies at present.

SCC pp 135–139

Q 11. What are the clinical features of a raised ICP?

A 11. Normal ICP is approximately 10 mmHg. Pressures over 40 mmHg are severely abnormal and associated with poorer outcomes. The ICP may remain normal until decompensation occurs.

Deterioration following head injury is almost always due to increased ICP. Increased ICP may be caused by either cerebral oedema or extra-cerebral compression (extradural or subdural haematomata).

Compression is usually associated with a progressive course, which may be rapid.

As well as neurological deterioration, other indications of raised ICP include pupillary dilatation, hemiparesis, hemiplegia and decerebration.

Raised ICP due to external compression requires rapid decompression and raised ICP due to cerebral oedema usually requires medical management with mannitol.

SCC pp 99–107

Q 12. How would you manage a patient with a spinal cord injury?

A 12. At the scene of accident it is necessary to maintain in-line spinal immobilisation which requires supporting of neck with stiff collar and sandbags and the patient should be transported on spinal board.

The *initial* priorities of hospital management of spinal injury patients remain ABC.

History
A spinal injury should be suspected if any major accident, unconscious patient, fall from a height, sudden jerk of neck after rear end car collision, facial injuries or head injury. Directly ask about neck or back pain, numbness, tingling, weakness, ability to pass urine.

Examination

- Primary survey
  - Intubation if necessary requires maintenance of in-line immobilisation.
  - Pharyngeal stimulation with airway can cause vagal discharge and cardiac arrest.
  - Cervical spine injuries reduce sympathetic outflow.
  - Patients may be both hypotensive and bradycardic (not a feature of hypovolaemia therefore suspect spinal cord injury).
  - Aggressive fluid resuscitation can induce pulmonary oedema.
- Secondary survey
  - Logroll – look for bruising, palpate for a step, tenderness.
  - Repeated neurological examination to determine neurological damage and its progression/resolution.
  - Systematic examination for fractures as patient may not feel pain.
  - In tetraplegic patients respiratory failure may be due to intercostal paralysis, partial phrenic nerve palsy, impaired ability to cough or a ventilation-perfusion mismatch.
  - In paraplegic patients respiratory failure may be due to variable intercostal nerve paralysis or associated chest injuries.
  - May develop as a late feature due to ascending oedema in the cervical cord.
  - Abdomen may be flaccid with absence of sensation (features of peritonism may be absent).
  - Priapism may develop.

Imaging

- X-rays – Cervical spine AP, lateral including C7/T1 (swimmers view or pull arms down to visualise), open mouth view of odontoid peg. AP and lateral view of other tender areas of spine. Image the entire spine if a spinal fracture is present.
- CT scan shows bony injury, magnetic resonance imaging (MRI) scan shows soft tissue involvement.

If neurological damage:

- Insert a urinary catheter.
- Note reduced BP and bradycardia due to neurogenic shock. Exclude hypotension due to haemorrhage elsewhere.
- Invasive monitoring is required.
- Give methylprednisolone intravenous 30 mg/kg over 15 minutes then 5.4 mg/kg/hr for next 23 hours. Needs to be given within 8 hours. Discuss with local spinal injuries unit.
- Pressure area care – regular turning.

SCC pp 108–112

Q 13. What methods are employed to try to prevent multi-organ dysfunction syndrome (MODS)?

A 13. Prevention can be grouped into three broad time periods; the resuscitation phase, the operative phase and the intensive care phase.

Resuscitation	Along the lines of ATLS principles: Airway, breathing, circulation, with the objectives being to maintain organ perfusion and oxygenation.
Operative treatment	Early, appropriate operative intervention, with clear objectives. This is the safest way. A planned second procedure is often better than waiting until complications occur.
Intensive care unit (ICU) management	Standard ICU practice of ventilatory support, renal support, antibiotics that are appropriately targeted and appropriate nutrition.

SCC pp 112–116

Q 14. How would you manage a patient with a severe upper gastrointestinal bleed?

A 14. The principles are *resuscitate*, *investigate* and then *endoscopy*.

Resuscitation takes the form of circulatory support with two large-bore cannulae, and fluid therapy with crystalloid or transfusion. Normal saline should be avoided in patients with suspected liver disease.

Investigations include haemoglobin which may remain normal until haemodilution occurs, urea and electrolytes (urea is elevated in severe bleeds), cross-match, liver function tests and prothrombin time.

Endoscopy should be performed on the next list after resuscitation unless the bleeding is profuse. Non-variceal bleeding can be treated endoscopically using thermal probes, injection of epinephrine or sclerosants, clips, staples or sutures, or a combination.

Variceal bleeding can necessitate the insertion of a Sengstaken-Blakemore tube as a temporising measure. A transjugular intrahepatic portosystemic shunt (TIPSS) may be necessary.

Surgery is reserved for failure of endoscopic therapy.

SCC pp 129–131

Q 15. How would you manage a patient with blunt chest trauma?

A 15. The physiological consequences of blunt chest trauma are altered ventilatory mechanics, decreased oxygenation, increased shunting and painful breathing resulting in inhibition of coughing leading to sputum retention and decreased tidal volume.

The effects of the chest injury and these physiological changes are hypoxia and hypercarbia leading potentially to ARDS.

Treatment is aimed at preventing ARDS and reversing these physiological changes. Oedema is prevented by fluid restriction, physiotherapy can help prevent atelectasis. Oxygenation is increased by increasing F_IO_2.

Life threatening injuries such as tension or open pneumothorax, massive haemothorax and flail chest need to be excluded. This should be done during the primary survey. A chest radiograph will reveal most abnormalities.

During the secondary survey arterial blood gases should be measured and an electrocardiogram (ECG) is performed. Blunt cardiac and lung injuries should be sought. A chest tube should be considered for haemothoraces, pneumothoraces or any patient undergoing positive pressure ventilation or aerial evacuation.

Analgesia for rib fractures will facilitate breathing.

SCC pp 146–151

Q 16. **What is systemic inflammatory response syndrome (SIRS) and how would you diagnose it?**

A 16. The systemic inflammatory response syndrome (SIRS) is a protective response by the body to attack from pathogens or other insult resulting in tissue damage. Positive feedback perpetuates the response leading to an unopposed inflammatory state giving the typical clinical picture of SIRS. The primary precipitating event results in tissue injury through infection, trauma, tumour invasion, hypoxia or ischaemia.

The main causes are:

- Localised or generalised sepsis
- Peritonitis (especially associated with pancreatitis)
- Burns
- Trauma
- Haemorrhage (particularly when associated with hypotension and hypoperfusion)

There then follows a secondary inflammatory response. The immune system is alerted to the threat posed by the tissue damage and reacts by instituting an inflammatory response to protect the body. This becomes exaggerated and subject to repeated positive feedback, leading to uncontrolled propagation by the inflammatory mediators involved. This results in endothelial cell damage and breakdown, causing the detrimental effects observed in SIRS.

This cascade involves several inflammatory mediators which are represented in *Table 3.4*.

Table 3.4 Inflammatory Mediators in SIRS

Cytokines	Arachidonic acid derivatives	Stress hormones	Other mediators
Tumour Necrosis Factor (TNF)	Prostaglandins	Catecholamines	Histamine
Interleukins (IL1, IL6)	Leukotrienes	Steroids	Serotonin
Platelet Activating Factor (PAF)	Thromboxanes	Insulin	Bradykinin

The diagnosis of SIRS is made by the patient fulfilling two or more of the following criteria:

- Core temperature >38°C or <36°C
- Heart rate (HR) >90/min
- Respiratory rate (RR) > 20/min or $PaCO_2$ < 4.26 kPa (32 mmHg)
- White cell count (WCC) >12 × 10^9/l or <4 × 10^9/l (with >10% neutrophils or immature forms)

Gastrointestinal tract (GIT) bacterial translocation and the transfer of endotoxin via the hepatic portal venous system may be an important factor as a constant triggering mechanism in the propagation of this exaggerated response.

Nitric oxide (NO) also referred to as endothelium-derived relaxing factor (EDRF) is involved in the tonic relaxation of vascular smooth muscle, opposing the myogenic contraction of the vessel walls. With the onset of SIRS, the homeostasis of vascular tone is altered, and NO mediated vasodilatation predominates, leading to the clinical effects seen in this condition.

Clinical effects of SIRS
These will vary depending on the precipitating cause and degree of involvement.

There may be:

- Overt or occult infection
- Flushed, warm peripheries
- Hypotension (particular diastolic)
- Tachycardia
- Hypoxia
- Metabolic acidosis on arterial blood gas (ABG) (due to hypoperfusion and lactic acid accumulation)
- Deranged clotting function (since the coagulation cascade may be involved in the inflammatory response)

SCC pp 112–116

Q 17. **What is MODS?**

A 17. Multi-organ dysfunction syndrome (MODS) is a progression from SIRS, resulting in end-organ dysfunction. It is diagnosed by dysfunction of two or more organ systems. The inflammatory process results in hypoperfusion and ischaemia of the tissues. The clinical picture will depend on the organ systems affected.

Respiratory
Often involved since they receive all of the cardiac output. Acute lung injury (ALI) and ARDS may occur following SIRS. The patient will be hypoxic, and show signs and symptoms of respiratory failure.

Cardiovascular
Endothelial damage leads to extraversation of fluid from the vessels into the interstitium resulting in oedema. Vasodilatation of arteries and veins result in hypotension, with tissue hypoxia and lactic acidosis. There may be myocardial dysfunction resulting from the direct effects of inflammation on the heart and circulating mediators or endotoxin (in sepsis).

Renal
There is oliguria (<0.5 ml/kg/hr of urine production) because of reduced renal perfusion and filtration of inflammatory matter. Urea and creatinine may be elevated.

Hepatic
Hypoperfusion results in reduced metabolism of drugs and hormones, poor control of glucose homeostasis, synthetic failure e.g. coagulation factors and failure to conjugate bilirubin (jaundice). The immunological role of the liver may be compromised; reducing the ability to detoxify translocated bacteria from the GIT, thereby worsening SIRS. Tests of extrinsic coagulation and liver function may be abnormal.

GIT
Hypoperfusion and ischaemia results in atrophy. This increases the risk of bacterial translocation, thereby continuously triggering the inflammatory response.

Cerebral
There may be confusion, sedation or agitation.

Haematological
There may be anaemia, thrombocytopenia, leucopenia, or leucocytosis. The tests of coagulation may show a range of

abnormalities from prolonged intrinsic (APPT) and extrinsic (PT) clotting times to frank disseminated intravascular coagulopathy (DIC).

If MODS is allowed to continue unchecked then the organ dysfunction will become irreversible. At this stage, multi-organ failure is said to have occurred. This progression is potentially avoidable with appropriate treatment.

SCC pp 112–116

Q 18. What are the principles of management in MODS?

A 18. The treatment aims are to support the organ-systems affected, and improve tissue perfusion and oxygenation.

Optimisation of oxygen delivery (DO_2) to the tissues:

$$DO_2 = CO \times (1.34 \times Hb \times {}^{Sat}/_{100}) + \text{dissolved fraction}$$

where CO (cardiac output) = SV $\times$ HR and BP = SVR $\times$ CO
dissolved fraction = $(PaO_2 \times 0.003)$

DO_2 can be maximised by maintaining adequate:

- Preload – fluid optimisation to increase stroke volume (SV).
- Afterload – α-agonists to increase systemic vascular resistance (SVR).
- Inotropic function – β-agonists to increase SV.
- Chronotropic function – β-agonists to increase HR.
- Haemoglobin concentration – this should be maintained above 10 g/dl.
- Haemoglobin saturation should be maintained above 94%. This may require mechanical ventilation.

Searching for and treating sources of sepsis:

These may be the primary precipitating cause responsible for SIRS or secondary colonisation, particularly in an immunocompromised host. Despite the active inflammatory response, the body's ability to deal with active infection is often low. The use of routine antibiotics cannot be recommended. Frequent tissue samples should be cultured and antimicrobial therapy directed at positively identified pathogens.
In overwhelming or partially treated infection, positive cultures may be impossible to isolate. Blind therapy should be instituted

only with the close involvement of the microbiology department. Inappropriate therapy may generate resistant strains and make further treatment difficult.

Maintain adequate urine output (>0.5 ml/kg/hr):

This will require careful fluid titration, often with invasive monitoring of central venous pressure (CVP or PAOP). Haemofiltration may be required.

Prevention of malnutrition:

These patients are catabolic and have increased energy requirements, their increased substrate demand should be reflected in nutritional regimens.

The aim of the treatment outlined above is to avoid progression to multi-organ failure syndrome (MOFS), which is a progression from MODS. This implies that irreversible damage has been done to the organ systems affected causing them to fail.

Prognosis
The risk of mortality depends on many factors (*Table 3.5*):

- Age
- Pre-morbid health
- Severity of disease
- The presence of sepsis
- Number of organ systems affected and the duration of failure

Table 3.5 Mortality rates in MOFS

Number of failed organ systems	Mortality on 1st day of organ failure	Mortality on 4th day of organ failure
2	50%	65%
3	80%	95%

SCC pp 112–116

Q 19. **What are the advantages and disadvantages of enteral nutrition?**

A 19. Enteral nutrition can take many forms:

- Oral supplements
- Enteral tube feeding

— Nasogastric
— Nasojejunal
— Percutaneous gastrostomy (PEG) (unusual in the critically ill)
— Percutaneous jejunostomy (PEJ) (usually after surgery)

Advantages

■ Cheap and simple to implement
■ No central venous access required
  — ↓ risk of infection
  — ↓ risk of mechanical complications of insertion
■ Maintains the physiological role of the GIT
■ Improved GIT blood flow:
  — prevents breakdown of mucosal lining
  — prevents translocation of GIT bacteria
  — prevents the development of SIRS and MODS

■ Protects against stress ulceration
■ Early commencement (within the first 24 hours)
  — ↓ ICU stay
  — ↓ septic complications
  — particularly true in multi-trauma

Disadvantages

■ Need functioning GIT
■ ↑ risk of nosocomial pneumonia
■ Delivery system (tubes) are source of morbidity:
  — Nasal ulceration
  — Sinusitis
  — Traumatic removal (poorly tolerated by some patients)
  — Tube occlusion
  — Displaced tubes
  — Peritonitis with percutaneous tubes
  — Bacterial colonisation
■ Lower oesophageal sphincter (LOS) dysfunction can lead to regurgitation and aspiration of feed
■ ↑ incidence of diarrhoea
■ ↑ incidence of nausea and vomiting
■ Malabsorption leads to malnourishment, which can be difficult to detect
■ Hyperglycaemia

SCC pp 140–146

Q 20. What are the advantages and disadvantages of parenteral nutrition?

A 20. Advantages

- All of prescribed feed reaches the bloodstream
- Rests damaged areas of the GIT
- Fluid input may be precisely recorded

Disadvantages

- Central venous access required
  - Invasive
  - expertise needed
  - infection risk
  - associated morbidity
- Expensive
- Unphysiological
  - fatty liver may result from lipid load
  - ↑ insulin requirements
- GIT atrophy
- No protection from stress ulceration

SCC pp 140–146

Q 21. How may nutrition regimens be tailored to patients with organ dysfunction?

A 21. Cardiac
Low Na^+ and low H_2O to decrease the risk of fluid overload and oedema production.

Respiratory
Aim to decrease the respiratory quotient (RQ) by increasing fat and reducing carbohydrate content. RQ is the amount of CO_2 produced per unit O_2 utilised. RQ for carbohydrate is 1 and 0.7 for fat. A high fat/low carbohydrate diet will reduce CO_2 production by the tissues, thereby decreasing the workload of the respiratory system.

Renal
Reduce protein content to decrease urea production in the liver. Renal patients also have poor handling of high fat diets. There should be reduced volume (↓H_2O and ↓Na^+) to prevent fluid

overload. Since they have a tendency towards hyperkalaemia K^+ should be avoided and monitored regularly.

Liver
Decreased H_2O and Na^+ content to prevent the development of fluid overload, particularly in patients with ascites. Nitrogen content should be lowered in encephalopathic patients. There should be an adequate carbohydrate load since there is a tendency towards hypoglycaemia, due to reduced glycogen storage.

Cerebral
Glucose is the main substrate in the brain. Close blood sugar control is required, as hyperglycaemia worsens cerebral oedema, and hypoglycaemia results in tissue damage.

Stressed patient have a tendency to hyperglycaemia due to the effects of adrenaline and noradrenaline on glucose handling. The 'fight' or 'flight' response liberates glucose from glycogen stores in preparation for action. Limit glucose to 5 g/kg/day. Insulin sliding scale may be required.

SCC pp 140–146

Q 22. **What are the daily nutritional requirements of patients and how may these vary with critical illness?**

A 22. This depends on:

■ Size which is assessed by body mass index (BMI) (also known as the Quatelet index)

$$BMI = \frac{Weight\ (kg)}{Height^2\ (m^2)}$$

— 20–25 is normal
— <19 is malnourished
— 25–30 is overweight
— 30–35 is obese
— >35 is morbidly obese
■ Pre-morbid nutritional status
■ Current clinical condition and metabolic demands

Daily requirements
These are divided into protein and non-protein (carbohydrate and fat) energy. The proportions of these will vary depending on

the individual needs of the patient. It should be noted that patients receiving infusions of propofol require less fat added to their feed.

$$\text{Nitrogen balance} = \text{Intake} - \text{Loss g N/day}$$

$$\text{Intake} = \frac{\text{Protein}}{6.25} \ (\text{g N/day})$$

Nitrogen requirement is 0.2 g/kg/day.

This is usually 9 g N/day for males and 7.5 g N/day for females.

- In non-catabolic patients, this represents 1 g N per 200 kcal energy
- In catabolic patients, this represents 1 g N per 80–100 kcal energy

Glutamine is an essential amino acid and it is important for wound healing and gluconeogenesis. It must be added to feed since it is unstable in solution.

Energy requirements are calculated from basal metabolic rate (BMR), this is usually 20–30 kcal/kg/day:

- 2500 kcal for males
- 2000 kcal for females

Table 3.6 Variability in energy requirements during critical illness

↑ *Energy requirements*	↓ *Energy requirements*
Patients being conscious, sitting or ambulatory	Patients being unconscious and sedated
Pyrexia	Mechanical ventilation
Malnutrition	
Sepsis and burns	

SCC pp 140–146

Q 1. What are the differences between sepsis, severe sepsis and septic shock?

A 1. Sepsis

The systemic response to infection manifested by two or more of the following:

- Temperature > 38 or <36°C
- Heart rate (HR) > 90 beats per minute
- Respiratory rate (RR) > 20 breaths per minute or hyperventilation $PaCO_2$ < 4.25 kPa
- WBC > 12 × 10⁹/l or <4 × 10⁹/l or >10% immature forms

Severe sepsis

Sepsis with organ dysfunction, hypoperfusion or hypotension (Systolic BP < 90 mmHg or a drop of more than 40 mmHg).

Septic shock

Defined as sepsis with hypotension, despite adequate fluid resuscitation, along with the presence of perfusion abnormalities.

SCC pp 163–165

Q 2. What are the features of occult intra-abdominal sepsis and how would you diagnose and treat it?

A 2. The clinical features are abdominal distension, pain, rebound, guarding and peritonism. Also, the presence of a mass, pyrexia (especially a swinging pyrexia), a metabolic acidosis, neutrophilia and thrombocytopenia.

Diagnosis can be assisted by ultrasound and computerised tomography (CT) but essentially is surgical through a laparotomy. Swabs and samples should be sent for culture including blood, urine, faeces, abdominal drain fluid and any rectal or vaginal discharge.

Treatment is laparotomy (this can be a diagnostic procedure). Antibiotics should be appropriately targeted with microbiological advice. Radiological drainage may be appropriate under either ultrasonic or CT guidance.

Q 1. **What are the principles for the safe transfer of the critically ill surgical patient?**

A 1. The principles for the safe transfer of the critically ill surgical patient are:

- Planning and communication between specialists at both referring and receiving units
- Experienced staff for the transfer – one experienced intensive therapy unit (ITU) doctor and one qualified ITU nurse/operating department practitioner (ODP)/technician
- Appropriate equipment and vehicle with good access, lighting and temperature control and a power supply for the relevant monitoring
- Full assessment and investigation prior to transfer – including electrocardiogram (ECG), arterial blood gas (ABG), central venous pressure (CVP), urine output and chest X-ray. A pneumothorax should be excluded prior to aerial transfer.
- Extensive monitoring that is robust, lightweight and battery powered
- Meticulous stabilisation of the patient including intubation prior to transfer. Vascular access should also be secure.
- Continual reassessment
- Continuing care during transfer – monitoring SaO_2, CO_2, heart rate (HR), temperature and intra-arterial blood pressure (non-invasive blood pressure is difficult to measure whilst in an ambulance or a helicopter)
- Direct handover
- Communication with relatives
- Documentation and audit

SCC pp 189–191

Q 2. **What are the basics of successful clinical monitoring of the critically ill patient?**

A 2. **Invasive and non-invasive measures**

For adequate monitoring the following tubes, lines and machines are necessary.

- Venous access – two large bore peripheral cannulae, venous cutdown or femoral lines, taking blood for haemoglobin, biochemical profile and cross-match
- Urinary catheterisation allowing monitoring of urine output
- ECG – monitoring for arrhythmias or ischaemia
- Pulse oximetry (transcutaneous estimation of oxygen saturation)
- Central venous catheterisation – CVP measurement
- Temperature measurement – core or peripheral

Clinical measurements

Standard clinical measurements include general appearance, respiratory rate (RR), pulse rate, blood pressure, urine output and CVP measurement.

Regular investigations

These include (but not exclusively) urea and electrolytes, haemoglobin, haematocrit, white cell count, ABG, temperature, pulmonary artery occlusion pressure and a sepsis check.

SCC pp 205–207

Q 3. **What parameters would make you consider early referral to critical care?**

A 3. Most hospitals have an early warning scoring system. An example is shown below. A score of three or more indicates a need to refer, but do not forget that trends are just as important as individual values.

	3	2	1	0	1	2	3
HR		<40	41–50	51–100	101–110	111–130	>130
Mean BP	<70	71–80	81–100	101–199		>200	
RR		<8		9–14	15–20	21–29	>30
Temp		<35	35.1–36.5		36.6–37.4	>37.5	
AVPU*				A	V	P	U

*A = Alert, V = Responds to verbal commands, P = Responds to pain, U = Unresponsive.

SCC pp 189–191

Q 4. **What are the principles of analgesia in the multiple injured patient?**

A 4. Analgesia should be adequate, appropriate and observed. It can be systemic or regional.

Adequate analgesia can facilitate breathing (rib fractures).

Appropriate analgesia is intravenous or intramuscular opioid initially. Non-steroidal anti-inflammatory drugs (NSAIDs) may also be appropriate acutely. Regional techniques are useful in some cases but may mask compartment syndrome and therefore liaison between specialities is essential. Patient controlled analgesia (PCA) is also a useful technique.

Monitoring of analgesic requirements is mandatory. If a patient's analgesic requirement suddenly increases then think why – is it infection, an occult injury or a developing compartment syndrome?

Systemic opioids should be given in small quantities frequently. An NSAID may reduce opioid requirements. Regional anaesthesia decreases respiratory depression.

Simple splintage of fractures will also reduce analgesic requirements.

SCC pp 203–205

Q 5. **What reasons might you want a surgical patient to go to intensive therapy unit (ITU) electively?**

A 5. The reasons are either for monitoring or for support. ABCDE is once again the mnemonic:

A   Airway monitoring for head and neck surgery
B   Breathing monitoring after cardiothoracic or upper abdominal surgery
C   Circulatory monitoring after cardiac and vascular surgery or in patients with cardiovascular disease
D   Disability monitoring after neurosurgery
E   Elective ventilation following cardiac or major abdominal surgery

The management plan should be formulated between both anaesthetist and surgeon. Adequate re-warming and analgesia should be ensured and blood should be monitored.

SCC pp 189–191

Q 6. What is meant by scoring systems for intensive care unit (ICU) patients? What scoring systems do you know?

A 6. The principle aim of intensive care is to provide the highest level and best quality of care available. This will involve evaluating the outcome after ICU treatment, which is difficult for this group of patients. The most frequently used determinant of successful treatment is the hospital mortality rate (which is the death rate before discharge from hospital of patients who have been treated in ICU). This does not take into account the quality of life thereafter for the patient or their family.

The aim of scoring systems used clinically is to evaluate outcome for different groups of ICU patients. These may be used to:

■ Determine different patient groups according to the severity of illness
■ Attach risk to each different group:
— For mortality rate (survivability)
— For division into separate groups for clinical trials
■ Compare different ICUs in different hospitals

These scoring systems **do not** predict outcome or guide treatment planning for individual patients.

Problems with scoring systems

1. Risk adjustment takes into account the differences between patients that affect their risk of any particular outcome, which is independent of the care that they receive. Risk is increased by:
   ■ Increasing age
   ■ Significant pre-morbid illness
   ■ The admitting diagnosis
   ■ The severity of the presenting illness
   ■ Emergency surgery

These factors constitute the case mix, and case mix adjustment is the process of accounting for these in the determination and comparison of any outcome measure (usually the hospital mortality rate).

2. Selection bias is an error in the predictive power if the database population differs from the sample population, i.e. it has to be validated for that population.

3. Lead-time bias is the effect of treatment (including treatment duration) on the patient before entering the ICU.
4. There needs to be a complete and accurate data set to prevent errors from multiplying.

The commonly used ICU scoring systems are:

APACHE	**A**cute **P**hysiology **a**nd **C**hronic **H**ealth **E**valuation
SAPS	**S**implified **A**cute **P**hysiology **S**core
MPM	**M**ortality **P**robability **M**odels

These systems assign different scores (weighting) to the measured variables. Scores are not only applied to assess severity of illness, but also severity of traumatic injury sustained. Those commonly used include:

- Revised trauma score (RTS) – this correlates well with survival. An RTS of 12 is associated with 99.5% survival, 6 with 63% survival and 0 with 3.7% survival
- Injury severity scale (ISS) – scores seven body areas from 1 (minor) to 5 (critical)
- Abbreviated injury score (AIS) – this is calculated from the sum of the squares of the three highest categories from the ISS. From this AIS score, the lethal dose in 50% (LD 50) has been calculated as:
  — 40 (ages 15–44)
  — 29 (ages 45–64)
  — 20 (age > 65)

SCC pp 198–201

Q 1. **What are the complications of inserting an intercostal chest drain?**

A 1. The complications are:

- Damage to thoracic or abdominal structures – this is almost universally done by inserting the chest tube with a trocar
- Infection (empyema)
- Neurovascular damage
  - Bleeding leading to haemothorax
  - Intercostal neuritis
- Incorrect tube position
  - Extra-pleural
  - Sub-diaphragmatic
- Tube complication
  - Blockage
  - Dislodgement
  - Disconnection
- Persistent pneumothorax
  - Large primary leak
  - Incomplete seal at skin
  - Inadequate underwater seal
- Subcutaneous emphysema
  - Leak through parietal pleura but not through skin

SCC pp 221–223

Q 2. **What are the indications for tracheostomy and what are its advantages?**

A 2. Major indications are airway obstruction, protection of the tracheo-bronchial tree and ventilatory insufficiency. Airway obstruction can be due to trauma (e.g. severe maxillo-facial trauma, severe head injury or severe facial burns), infection (acute epiglottitis) or oedema. Protection of the tracheo-bronchial tree is necessary for airway control after major oropharyngeal surgery, or following supraglottic surgery or head injury. Tracheostomy is useful for ventilatory insufficiency for prolonged ventilation (>2 weeks) e.g. severe chest trauma, coma or pulmonary diseases. Miscellaneous indications for tracheostomy include to decrease anatomic dead space, to facilitate tracheo-bronchial lavage and to assist in ventilator weaning.

Advantages of tracheostomy include decreased dead space, decreased work of breathing, decreased sedative requirements, increased efficiency of suctioning, it allows speaking and eating, weaning is quicker and intensive therapy unit (ITU) stay is decreased.

SCC pp 217–220

Q 3. **Describe how you would perform a venous cut-down of the long saphenous vein at the ankle.**

A 3. Venous cut-down is principally used for emergency vascular access in the trauma situation. It may also be used when central venous access is impossible. Any large vein is suitable although the long saphenous vein at the ankle is the favoured site.

The technique is similar for all sites.

A transverse skin incision is made 2 cm anterior and superior to the medial malleolus. The vein is dissected free by blunt dissection. Two ties are placed around the vein, the distal one secured tightly, and the proximal loose. A ventomy is performed. Insert a large 14G cannula into the venotomy and flush the cannula with 0.9% NaCl. The cannula is secured by tightening the upper ligature.

SCC pp 216–217

Q 4. **What are the findings for a diagnostic peritoneal lavage (DPL) to be positive?**

A 4. Diagnostic peritoneal lavage (DPL) detects free intraperitoneal blood with 97% accuracy. A positive test is indicated by any of the following:

- >10 ml frank blood
- ≥ 100,000 RBC/ml

- ≥ 500 WBC/ml
- Bile/Bowel contents drained from catheter
- Gram stain positive for bacteria
- Peritoneal lavage fluid drained from catheter or chest tube

False positive results may arise from haemorrhage from the surgical incision or from bleeding from pelvic fractures.

SCC pp 223–225

Q 5. **Why might you consider monitoring intra-abdominal pressure (IAP)?**

A 5. Intra-abdominal pressure (IAP) is an important measure of underlying abdominal problems and an indicator of a patient's physiological status. Monitoring of IAP in the critically ill is gaining favour. Slight increases in IAP have been shown to have deleterious effects on organ function.

Clinical importance of IAP:

- IAP greater than 10 mmHg has been demonstrated to be instrumental in organ dysfunction. Intra-abdominal hypertension (IAH) > 25 mmHg is deleterious to both intra- and extra-abdominal organs. IAH is an independent risk factor for intensive care unit (ICU) mortality and has been demonstrated in 30% of a surgical ICU population.
- Raised IAP affects chest wall mechanics and decompression has beneficial effects on respiratory mechanics and oxygenation.

SCC pp 228–229

Q 6. **What is a chest drain and how does it function?**

A 6. A chest drain is a conduit to remove air or fluid (blood, pus or a pleural effusion) from the pleural cavity. It allows re-expansion of the underlying lung and prevents the entry of air or drained fluid back into the chest. A chest drain must therefore have three components, it must be unobstructed, have a collecting container below chest level and a one-way mechanism such as water seal or Heimlich valve.

Mechanism of action:

Drainage occurs during expiration when pleural pressure is positive. Fluid within pleural cavity drains into the water seal through which air bubbles. The length of drain below the fluid level is important: more than 2–3 cm increases resistance to air drainage.

SCC pp 221–223

Q 7. **What are the indications and potential complications of central venous cannulation?**

A 7. The Indications are:

- Monitoring of central venous pressure (CVP)
- Fluid infusion
- Drug infusions (most inotropes have to be given centrally)
- Blood sampling
- PA catheter insertion
- Triphosphopyridine nucleotide (TPN)
- Haemofiltration
- Transvenous cardiac pacing
- Chemotherapy
- No possibility of peripheral venous access

Complications:

- Pneumothorax/haemothorax (more common with subclavian or low internal jugular approaches)
- Arterial puncture (can be catastrophic with subclavian artery rupture since there is no way to occlude this vessel)
- Nerve injury
  - Phrenic, vagus and sympathetic chain in the neck
  - Femoral nerve in the groin
- Cardiac arrhythmias
- Air embolus with neck cannulation in hypovolaemic patients
- Erosion through vessel wall (including myocardium)
- Formation of A-V fistula
- Thoracic duct injury in the neck (with left sided cannulation)
- Infection:
  - Use careful aseptic technique for insertion
  - Avoid sites with skin erythema
  - TPN increases the risk of infection and should be infused via a dedicated line. Sites should be changed regularly (every 5–7 days)

Practical Procedures

Answers

- Ectopic placement – this is not always avoidable but should be recognised:
  — Ensure that free aspiration of blood is possible
  — Check position with CXR

Contra-indications to insertion:

- Bleeding diatheses (especially with the subclavian route, since occlusion of a bleeding vessel is more difficult)
- Localised infection

These are relative and clinical need must be considered for each individual case.

SCC pp 211–214

Q 8. **Outline the relevant anatomy of a) the internal jugular vein (IJV) and b) the subclavian vein. Describe the technique used to cannulate each of these central veins.**

A 8. **Internal jugular vein (IJV)**
Anatomy:

- The IJV is formed from the jugular bulb, which drains blood from the brain via the sigmoid sinus.
- It passes through the jugular foramen and then follows a straight line to the sternoclavicular joint, where it joins the subclavian vein to form the brachiocephalic vein.
- The IJV is intimately associated with the internal carotid artery throughout its course – initially posterior and finally antero-lateral to it.
- The IJV, internal carotid artery and vagus nerve all travel within the carotid sheath.
- The IJV is superficial in the upper part of its course, covered by the sternomastoid muscle in the middle part and splits the sternal and clavicular heads of that muscle in the lower part.

Cannulation technique:

- Head down position
- Clean skin
- Infiltrate with local anaesthetic
- A syringe should be attached to needle at all times to reduce the risk of pneumothorax
  — Mid/high approach – lateral to carotid artery at the level of the cricoid cartilage

— Low approach – between the heads of sternomastoid (reduced risk of arterial puncture but increase risk of pneumothorax)

■ Insert the needle, and advance aiming towards the ipsilateral nipple
■ Once blood is aspirated continue with the Seldinger technique

Subclavicular vein (SCV)
Anatomy:

■ Continuation of the axillary vein
■ Runs from the lateral border of the first rib, and arches upwards over the rib
■ It's most cephalad point is at the mid-clavicular line
■ Joins the IJV to form the brachiocephalic vein behind the sternoclavicular joint
■ The external jugular vein drains into SCV

Cannulation technique:

■ Head down position
■ Clean skin
■ Local anaesthetic infiltration
■ A syringe should be attached to needle at all times to reduce the risk of pneumothorax
■ The needle is inserted at the mid-clavicular line or junction of medial third and lateral two thirds of clavicle
■ 'Walk off' the clavicle aiming towards the suprasternal notch
■ Once blood is aspirated continue with the Seldinger technique

Seldinger technique:

■ Needle with syringe attached
■ Once blood is freely aspirated, detach the syringe and feed the guide wire (with the flexible J tip first) for approximately 15 cm
■ Remove the needle (taking care not to displace wire)
■ Extend the skin incision with a scalpel blade
■ Advance the dilator over the wire (and remove)
■ Insert the catheter over the wire
■ Remove the wire
■ Aspirate blood and flush all lines with heparinised saline
■ CXR to confirm position

SCC pp 211–214